Will My Belly Button Ever Look the Same Again?

My Pregnancy Journal

LESLIE ANDERSON

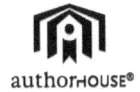

authorHOUSE®

AuthorHouse™
1663 Liberty Drive, Suite 200
Bloomington, IN 47403
www.authorhouse.com
Phone: 1-800-839-8640

First published by AuthorHouse 8/27/2007

ISBN: 978-1-4343-2867-0 (sc)

Printed in the United States of America
Bloomington, Indiana

This book is printed on acid-free paper.

Cover design by Jenn Taylor.

Contents

It's Official!!

Well... :) The test at the doctor's came out positive! I knew it! My dear bf finally believes it and we have 9 months to get everything together and have the perfect Christmas with our new baby!

I still haven't told anyone. I'm nervous. Maybe I'll tell them after the first sono... I don't know! Even though I'm already 28, I'm still the first of my college friends to get pregnant! And we're not married yet. eek... I'm happy but I'm afraid that I won't be as close with all of them. Ah well, they'll be joining me soon enough, I'm sure.

I'll write more later. I've gotta go you-know-where to do you-know-what...

So Bigmouth (My Bf) Told Everyone...

My boyfriend could not keep the happy news to himself, so he told his father. Then his father told his mother (they don't even live together!). He said he was just talking "man-to-man" and didn't mean for his father to actually leak the news.

I'm only what, 4, 5 weeks along! I barely feel pregnant! I just feel like I'm a little bit tired (okay I slept until noon today, but that's because I was up all night peeing and drinking water). But I mean- I guess I'm still in disbelief so I really don't want to tell anyone.

I told my mother. Now I have to tell my father.

1

I'm worried. Is it too early to tell people? I'm just telling my family so far.

Oh yeah, bf has decided on the name Georgia (nickname Georgie after his grandmother) if it's a girl. I don't know. It's different. It's easy to spell. Those are two good reasons. But every time I say it I hear the song playing in my head. That would get old after a few months, years, decades... I don't know.

2006-04-25 (5 weeks)

Should I Be Worried?

Okay. So I still don't feel pregnant yet. I don't have any morning sickness yet. I felt a little light-headed this morning but I was fine after I sat down for a minute. My boobs aren't any bigger yet. They're jigglier (?) but not any bigger. Maybe I'll just have little jiggle boobs. Hopefully my kid won't starve with these little things...

My only symptoms seem to be fatigue and gas, which, I mean- I had those things sometimes pre-pregnancy.

Anyway, everything is going fine, I guess. I just started working again this week! I get so tired at work! How does everyone handle this? I want to go to bed now, but my boyfriend asked me ever so nicely if I could make something for dinner. I told him that I'd try. I don't feel as sleepy as I did yesterday, so I should be able to whip something up.

At work, they have a hot chocolate machine... mmm... They also have individual coffee packs that you can brew in your own cup! Too bad I'm off of coffee. Oh well, I hope the hot chocolate wasn't too bad for me because I drank a whole cup. It helped me wake up a little bit. But then the afternoon dragged on...

So, what are some good things to eat for meals? This morning for breakfast I couldn't really eat but I drank most of a Nouriche smoothie and a piece of whole-wheat bread. Then at lunch I ate a turkey sandwich on whole-wheat with some yogurt and snacked on an orange a little bit later. For dinner I think we're having chicken flautas.

Speaking of dinner... I'd better get on it! Thanks to everyone for signing my journal! I'll write back one day when I'm not in a half-asleep, rambling mood.

Leslie

So I Told (Some) of My Friends

I told some of my friends yesterday when we went shopping at an outlet mall. I said- guys, I'm looking for new pants because I'm pregnant. They were really surprised.

I don't know what they think about it. At 28, I'm the first of my college buddies to get pregnant. And I'm not married yet. I think it was kind of a shocker. One of them asked if it was planned- I said... Well... I don't know.

That's a hard one to answer!! I guess if I could plan everything out ideally I'd be rich (maybe not rich but comfortable) and married and have a house with a dog. It's just so weird! Like my family and my boyfriend's family all think it's totally normal to start a family right now with everything up in the air (kinda, not really crazy in-the-air) but my friends are just a teensy bit freaked out about it. I think. They are a little excited to throw a baby shower.

It's just weird because I realized that I kind of feel alone in all of this. (I know I have all the people on here...) I freaked out a little bit this morning! Am I ready for a baby? What am I going to do??? I've got my degree but I don't have a "real" job yet. Should I get my "real" job (teaching)? Or should I wait another year until I'm settled in with the baby? If I started teaching in August, I'd have to leave to have the baby in December and probably come back to a crazy situation after my maternity leave.

Is it too much to have a first pregnancy and a first year of teaching? I know there are women out there who have done all that and more, but could I do it?

Well as far as my physical state- I'm doing great. I don't have much nausea, just a little when I try to wake up at 5 in the morning to pack lunches. I eat saltines and drink ginger ale a lot. I think they say the nauseous feeling is from your digestive system slowing down to absorb all of the nutrients- that's what also causes constipation! Well, as uncomfortable as that it, I think it's kind of amazing the way your whole body works for the baby. It's really kind of incredible. My friends really need to hop on this baby bandwagon! They don't know what they're missing! (Of course, if people don't want to have kids, they definitely shouldn't have them, you know?)

Anyway, enough rambling. Baby- you'd better be growing down there!!

I Feel Really Sick

Well, here I am at work and I feel sick to my stomach. I don't feel like I'm going to puke or anything. I feel like I just need to lie down. It's not helping matters much that there is very little work for me to do today. I'm very tempted to ask if I can leave early. Ugh! I need to hang in there because I know this is just the beginning (of the pregnancy, I mean).

As fatigued as I am feeling, when I get home from work, I just feel like eating and getting in the bed. So now my boyfriend thinks I'm mad at him! Ugh! That really does make me mad! :) He needs to understand that I have nothing against him- I'm just really really tired. I feel like I try my hardest to wake up at 5, send him off to work with a nice lunch, send myself off to work, come home, whip something up for dinner and clean up. So when he rambles on to me about some sports thing about pros against joes, I do my best to listen but PLEASE LET ME SLEEP some time or another. Whew!

Enough complaining, I guess. The good side in all of this is that we'll have extra money with both of us working so much. Maybe I'll be able to get a nice new safe car before the baby gets here. I'm even riding the bus to save on gas and parking so I'll get the car sooner. And a rocking chair. I'm working hard so I can buy a rocking chair. Does a regular rocking chair work on carpet, I wonder? Or will I have to buy one of those glider things?

Back to work!

Feeling a Little Lonely...

So I feel kinda lonely. I don't know why. I feel like I'm going through all of this nausea and everything alone. I'm just being pregnant I guess. I told my boyfriend all of this last night and he's trying to figure out what he can do. I don't know. There's nothing he can really do for me medically or anything of course. I told him just to be there. When I'm nauseous just give me a hug and tell me I'll be fine. You know. Let me know that he cares that I'm going through all of this. I read in my What to Expect book that one of the first trimester symptoms is having misgivings. I wonder exactly what that means and I wonder if that is what I'm feeling?

Physically, I'm still feeling okay. I feel a little tired. I feel a little achiness on my right side of my abdomen and I don't know what that's about. I'm sure if it was serious, it'd feel more painful. I'm at work and I just made it through half of the day- whew-hew! 4 hours left and I can go home and put on sweat pants. :)

I'm eating more. I find that it helps to munch all day instead of trying to eat a big meal. I think that it probably helps with my tummy problems too.

Back to work!

Feeling Better!!

So Friday I missed work because I felt sooo sick... I'm mean, not puking or anything, but I felt so nauseous, I'd figure I'd stay home. You know? I'm not trying to stress myself out or anything. I'm just working a little temp job to make some money for when the baby comes. I think I'm putting my career on hold for another year. I think. I can't imagine starting my first year of teaching in my third trimester. I know there are women who have done more, but oh well. I'm just trying to do what's best for me. I'm not superwoman or anything. So anyways. I'm sure years from now I'll appreciate this year off.

So Friday I felt sick sick sick... And I slept all weekend. My boyfriend's mom came over yesterday (mother's day!!) and he cooked everyone dinner. Everyone kept wishing me happy mother's day! Weird, huh??? Mother's Day... it was great. My own mother was off in Denver with our family for their family reunion. I missed it. Oh well. I'm mostly upset about all the good food I'm sure they had. Mmm-mmm... But I need to stay home and save money for the baby. Plus I'm flying out to Maryland to visit my mother next month sometime. I'm also going to try on bride's maid's dresses for my best friend's wedding!! It's going to be June of 2007. Hopefully by then I'll be back to my normal size??? I don't know!! Should I go ahead and order bigger just in case??? Who knows- maybe I'll have big huge boobs for the rest of my life (doubt it!!)

Right now I haven't really gained any weight I don't think. I may have lost weight since I was feeling so icky. Now that I'm feeling better I'll probably be eating like a pig! I don't know. Overeating gives me gas and hiccups and everything else so I don't think I'll ever have a problem with overeating. My boyfriend says I have gained a little weight in my lower stomach area- the baby area, not my jelly roll area... He kept thinking that the jelly roll area was the baby and I said, well, that's all me... The baby might be pushing it up, but that's all me. :) So today he says, you're gaining weight down there. Well, hmph! That's probably why my jeans don't fit! Everything else fits except the jeans.

anyway, back to why I started this. So today I still am very tired. I still feel achy in weird places. My back already hurts! Imagine when I'm toting an extra 30 pounds... jeez luweez... But I did not feel nauseous!! Hopefully the nausea is letting up a little bit! I hope I hope I hope! I know that other people on here celebrated the end of morning sickness a little too early, only to have it come back with a vengeance the next day or so later. I hope that's not me! I know that with my wacky stomach I'll probably have gas and heartburn all the way through, but as long as the nausea gives me a break, I think I'll be okay.

I'd better get off of here and cook dinner! I haven't cooked for my poor sweetie in weeks!

2006-05-23 (9 weeks)

Weird Symptoms

As soon as one thing quits, another thing starts! So finally my nausea seems to be gone but I have a lot of other weird things going on! I felt dizzy for a few days after the nausea went away. Then I started having a racing heart... weird... I read that it is normal, but I'm definitely writing that on the list to ask my doctor about!

I continue to be very very tired. I think today is the most tired I have been. I feel like I'm going to fall asleep at my desk! In fact, I'm going to put my head down for a few minutes before I have to get back to work.

Nausea Again???

This journal must be soooo boring to anyone that comes across it. :) But oh well. I'd like to remember this wacky first trimester stuff for the next time I decide to have a baby. Although, I'm beginning to understand why some people only have one baby!!

I've been sick for the past two days with some weird cold/flu thing. I felt like I had a cold, but I didn't have any coughing or congestion. I felt like I had the flu because I ached all over but I didn't have a fever. It was weird. I thought it was another weird side effect of pregnancy. I had a headache for like 3 days... I know that sounds terrible but since I was prone to headaches before pregnancy, I wasn't really worried about it. I felt like a real weakling! But you know what??? I didn't take a dang thing, not even a tylenol. I toughed it out! I did miss work, but I wanted to rest so maybe the baby wouldn't catch on that mommy was sick. I kept eating everything that my dear bf fed me even though I wanted to gag constantly.

So anyway, I get back to work after having missed two days. Talk about a short week, we had Monday off for Memorial Day, I worked Tuesday and now I'm back on Friday. It's almost 1 o'clock so I'm thinking maybe I'll make it through the whole day!

I get back to work today, and it turns out that most of the office had this weirdo bug this week. Not everyone missed as much work as I did, but I felt better knowing I wasn't just some pregnant weakling. I really thought it was all in my head, like I was stressing out or something.

I feel better, still a little achy, but better. Now I have to figure out what I'm going to do with my bf's six-year-old son all day tomorrow and Sunday! Ugh! I still need to recover! What's the poor kid gonna do while I'm stuck on the couch?

2006-06-05 (11 weeks)

Belly Button Changes

My belly button looks different!! The other night I was looking in the mirror and I realized that I could see the bottom of my belly button as plain as day. Usually it just looks like a deep dark hole, but now you can see right into it! Weird! Will my belly button ever look the same again??? I'll have to remember this. When my kids grow up I'll say- "kids, before I got pregnant my belly button looked entirely different from now..."

Of course I'm not just thinking about my belly button- I mean, what else is going to change about me? Physically, mentally? What things will remain changed and what will return back to normal? Will I still be the same person? It's all very interesting to think about.

2006-06-09 (12 weeks)

Significant Others

I need some ideas of what kinds of special things I can do for my boyfriend. I feel so terrible. He's been cleaning and cooking and doing everything while I just sit around or sleep. Last night he kept talking to me and I felt like I was going to fall asleep on my feet! He went in to take a shower and I don't remember anything after that except the back of my eyelids until 2 am when I woke up to go to the bathroom.

Anyway I wonder what I could do for him to let him know that I appreciate and love him? I've stopped cooking dinner, I've stopped packing his lunch- I don't run errands or go to the grocery store. Hell, I barely do my own laundry! Hopefully soon I'll get out of this funk but until then I wish I knew some little ways to let him know I love him.

2006-06-12 (12 weeks)

Feeling Better!! Yay!!

Okay so... This weekend I actually had enough energy to clean the house and cook dinner!!! I'm so excited. I did my laundry, even. :) I'm hoping this is a trend for the next couple of months.

I mean, don't get me wrong. I still have weird stuff going on with me. I have a backache that won't quit. I'm peeing even more frequently (didn't think it was possible). I'm still tired, but man, I was sooooo tired before. I was so tired it hurt- like my eye sockets hurt and my ears hurt and my neck hurt- just really really worn down. So hopefully I'm okay now for a few weeks or months.

gotta go. computers are down and work and I've been told to reboot...

So I'm back. The computers are still down at work. We've got internet access and not much else! So we're at a standstill. It's 1 o'clock and I'm getting ants in my pants! My dad and his girlfriend and my sister Kala are in town. I think they are just lounging around my house right now.

At least I'm getting paid for being here even though I am bored out of my skull! I've only got 4 hours left. Hopefully the computers will come back up so I can get _something_ done...

Heard the Heartbeat!!

Well I don't get to do an ultrasound until 20 weeks. I guess since I know exactly how far along I am, there's no need to do it. So, basically at the doctor, all I did was talk with the nurses and listen to the heartbeat.

It's awesome! So I guess there's really a baby in there, huh?

I also almost freaked out because I'm Rh negative. I guess just as a preventative measure they give me a shot (at 28 weeks I think?) in case the baby is Rh positive. I had no clue that only 5 to 10 percent of the population has O negative blood. That's so interesting.

Anyway, back to work...

Mood Swings

I guess I lashed out at my boyfriend yesterday. I used a lot of nasty language which isn't really like me! I think I was upset for a valid reason, but I feel bad for yelling and stuff.

I hope this isn't a new permanent side of myself. Hmph. Sometimes I don't know how to get my point across with him. I'm sure he listened last night! But he probably thinks I'm crazy now!

I don't know where my patience has gone.

2006-06-27 (14 weeks)

Movement

I can feel the baby move. I swear I've been feeling it for a few weeks now, but I haven't said anything because my boyfriend swears it's too early.

It's definitely movement and it's not gas. Feels like a little puppy wriggling around in there.

I'm supposed to make my next doctor's appointment today but I forgot all of the numbers at home. I guess that means I'll have to wait to do it until tomorrow!

2006-06-29 (14 weeks)

Told Everyone...

So I've finally told everyone. it's like really real... ya know! Like when I heard the heartbeat and I told the doctor- "well, I guess there's no denying there's something in there!!"

And my expanding waistline is undeniable too. I had to retire another pair of pants until post-pregnancy.

Well I'm off to bed. I'll write more some other time.

Don't You Hate...

So I went out to the mall to get something to eat and I saw the steak sandwich stand, and I was like- mmm... steak sandwich... I made a beeline for the steak sandwich stand and stood there while they chopped the meat and onions and such and grilled up my sandwich. So I sit down to eat. I get about halfway through the first half and I was like, "this tastes funny". My friends and my boyfriend were like, "is there something wrong with it? Do you want to take it back?" Nah, I think the spices just weren't agreeing with me. Sure enough, my dear bf tested it out and said the sandwich was fine. Baby just did not like it!!

How disappointing! To have a craving and spend like $7 on a combo (because we were downtown) only to end up not being able to eat it. Such is life!! It's funny though.

So I've been busy busy busy for a while. I made a last minute trip to see my dad. He and his girlfriend were very excited to see me and my little bump. So that was cool. We went to the 4th of July parade. It was alright... they usually have a flyover with military jets but I guess they were otherwise engaged for the day. It was nice to see a bunch of people though. I got to compare bellies with one of our family friends who is also pregnant. I think she's due in September though.

We're preparing the house for my 6-year old future stepson to move in with us. We moved the computer out to the dining room, so now my dear bf thinks the place looks like a cluttered old lady's apartment. Great. I don't know what we'll be able to do about that!

I've got to go eat lunch. I just wanted to catch up a bit.

Oh yeah! I forgot that I went maternity shopping yesterday with my friend Emily who is due in October. I bought the cutest blue shirt and some khaki capris. Her husband went with us and he was rather amused when, as we were leaving Babies R Us, we simultaneously handed him our bags and headed off to the potty. It was funny.

Babies R Us is a cool place. A bunch of preggos wondering around... kinda like this website!

2006-07-10 (16 weeks)

Oh Yeah! The Kicking!

I forgot to mention the kicking! I can really feel a lot of movement down there. Especially when I bend down like to pick something up by my feet. I was showing my boyfriend and he's like- "Because you're squishing its head!! That's why it's moving!!" :) Oh silly bf... The baby is kicking back in its little bag of water... squeezed? maybe. but squished? I don't think so.

He's still trying to feel the movement. He swears he feels it when I'm sleeping. But yesterday he was feeling my stomach and he said that something poked him back so he started talking to it. I told him I thought that he was a little far to the right and that gas bubbles hang out over there by my appendix. So he's like- "Great! So you're telling me I'm talking to a gas bubble?" I'm sure the baby could still hear him though.

2nd trimester rocks!!

Mommy Brain

So I'm beginning to figure out what the whole "Mommy brain" thing is... At first, I rejected the idea. hah! Losing your brainpower because of carrying a child... how preposterous! Now... I kinda realize that it's like teacher brain. It's not that you are dumber than you were previously. I think that you are just more preoccupied with things.

When I was student teaching there were always 10 different things that I was working on; 17 different kids that had owies or potty accidents or gum in their hair (or whatever...); 5 or 6 parents calling in at the last minute to remind me of something or other... I could go on and on... but if I forgot one thing (only to remember it at 6 pm after the day was over and I was headed home)... it's "uh-oh, little Jonathan is stranded somewheres because I forgot to tell him that he was supposed to wait for a ride instead of catch the bus..." That was like 3 years ago and it still haunts me to this day. I'm sure he's okay. It was my last day of student teaching. I never heard anything on the news or anything.

Anyway. :) So yesterday I was driving and spaced out because we were talking about baby names and I completely missed my turn that I've turned on a million times. But at the time I was in la-la baby land thinking of little pink bows and such. (watch it be a boy!)

And this morning! I completely dumped an entire cup of hot cocoa all over my lap. Like a huge puddle, dripping all over the place... and my brand new preggo pants are completely ruined. There's no getting rid of this huge huge stain, I'm sure. They kind of look like desert camo pants-maybe I should go for a new look?

Someone Please...

Please remind my boyfriend that "you're gonna be huge" is not a compliment!! :) He says "well, don't you want your baby to be big and fat? I love big and fat babies" Well. Not particularly, no. I mean, if it comes out and it's larger than average I'm not going to trade it in or anything, but jeez!! I'm only 17 weeks along and I already feel like the baby is getting a little bit big. I'm a small person! 5'1(&1/2)" I don't think there's any room down there for a big fat baby.

The baby just kicked again. She (or he or they) always kicks when I talk about her father. He can already feel the kicking so that's really cool. The other night he got to see what I saw one morning when I was laying on my back. Well, one morning I was laying on my back when he left for work and I could swear that I felt and saw the baby doing a somersault. Then the other night when we were watching tv I was propped up, but still on my back and it was like a huge ocean wave of baby popping up and wriggling around and I said "see!! look at that! She's flipping!" and of course he freaks out. He thinks that she (I know I know... watch it be a boy...) needs to quit or she's gonna strangle on her cord or something. I don't know. You'd think that if that were possible it would happen more often? I don't know. I think it's normal for them to flip like that when they're still small. Pretty soon she won't have any room to do anything in there at all.

But so anyways. Right before we went to bed that night or the next, I was laying on my back again and she starts doing it again but this time it really hurt! Dear bf thinks that means I should avoid sleeping on my back. And I have heard that in all of the books of course. I don't think I've ever actually slept on my back anyway. But if it's so unhealthy to be on your back then why do they put you on your back when you're at the doctor's?

So back to my dear bf. He really scared me that day when he talked about the baby strangling on her cord! I was okay after I felt her kicking a lot later in the day. I figure, well, if she's gonna flip, she's gonna flip, you know? I can't exactly ground her in-utero.

2006-07-20 (17 weeks)

18 Week Dr. Checkup- U/S Scheduled

I went to the doctor Tuesday night for a physical. Since I was transferring from the other place downtown they were really confused about what was going on with me... It took like 2 hours of waiting and the nurse midwife was only in there for like 15 minutes. It was 7 or so and she was ready to go home!! Well, they're the ones that offered me the 6 pm appointment, you know?? Bums. I still have more confidence in the people downtown. I'm giving this other place one more chance to get it together and I think I may switch back. I don't know. At least at this place you get to keep the same nurse midwife for every appointment. Downtown anyone can come in and see you. So anyway, apparently I have some sort of infection that I have to take some yucky antibiotics for. I hate taking medication, especially antibiotics! And it's making me so nauseous. It's got to be terrible for me, you know? I pray that it's not doing something weird to the baby. The directions say not to take it if you are in the first trimester or breast feeding!! I know that I'm in the second trimester, but man oh man... Hm... That just means that they can't link it to anything going wrong with the baby during the second and third trimester... That doesn't mean it can't do anything. I'm freaking out about that one. And the way it makes me sick to my stomach can't be good. I really feel like I'm going to lose my lunch.

And I wonder how that lady knows it's actually bacteria anyway? I mean, she took my pap smear, disappeared for an hour and presto chango she says I have a bacterial infection. I thought it was only bacteria if it grew on a petri dish. How did she do all that in an hour? Maybe things are more advanced since my high school science class. Who knows.

So anyway, I have my doubts. I just want to do what's best for the baby. I hope it's doing okay down there.

I heard the heartbeat again. It was great. I actually had been wondering about the baby after my hike back from the bus stop the other day. It was so hot... And when I got home I remembered that I left my keys at work (pregnancy brain!!) so I was locked out! It was really really hot... So I waited in the semi-cool hallway of our apartments for like 40 minutes because I thought dear bf was coming home soon. Then I hiked back to the bus stop to the CVS to call dear bf's sister. I bought a bottle of water and chugged that down and walked back home. I was feeling good. I thought to myself, well, if the doctor asks if I exercise, I can say heck yeah! But as I was reaching the home stretch, I could see the apartment and I only had a few more steps to go and I just felt one big cramp in my stomach, my thighs, my butt... ick! I felt sooo hot. I think I just had too much water all at once. In about 5 minutes dear bf was home and I sat down on the couch and I felt fine. I didn't even feel bad in the morning. The only thing is that the baby seemed to have slowed down his/her movements the entire next day. I don't know. The 'what to expect' book says that movements before 20 weeks can be unpredictable like that since the baby is so tiny. She (he) could have just been facing the rear and kicking at things I couldn't distinguish.

So I heard the heartbeat. I'm sure she's fine. First I boiled her for a little bit and now I'm giving her medicine that may or may not be safe... No more medicine after this!!

Oh yeah, the ultrasound is scheduled for August 9th! Then I'll find out if it's Aubrey or Joseph (I'm really over the name Georgia and I really haven't given boys names too much thought...)

2006-07-23 (18 weeks)

On Vacation

I'm just sitting here browsing journals like all of us do whenever we have a spare moment. It's amazing to me to see people on here that are due in April!! Wow! It just seems like yesterday that the December people were starting out their journals. And now... Wow, we're almost halfway through!! I can't believe it.

It's been great to be here at my mom's and be pregnant. I'm getting so spoiled and it's fun. Sorry to all of my friends out here! I'm only here for 4 days and I'm kinda just chillin' with my momma. Tomorrow I get to pick out bridesmaids' dresses with my best friend Christina and then on Tuesday I'm heading home.

Flying out here was very interesting!! I didn't have too many problems, but it is different being pregnant, I think. I don't know. It wasn't a major big deal, but it just felt different to be on a plane. My connection flight was sooooo screwed up! They kept changing the gate- it was so unreal. They could not decide which plane they were sending where!!! That's never happened to me before and it was soooo bizarre. We switched gates back and forth like 5 times and all of the electronic signs were all screwed up. There were people on our flight that didn't speak English and they were confused as heck! I couldn't imagine trying to figure that mess out travelling in another country. The airline people were telling us one thing and the signs said another. THEY ACTUALLY boarded and entire plane full of people and then like 30 minutes later had them get off of the plane and have everyone on my flight get on the plane. It was very very strange!! My brother says I should call the airline and get something free! :) Oh well- it really didn't bother me, really- to be honest. They only thing was, We were supposed to board at 1:00 and so I went to the bathroom like five minutes before that. But then we sat around for another hour and they never really told us when they were going to board, so I was kinda uptight about having time to pee before boarding. You know. I'm pregnant. I pee a lot.

Then. Then the flight was like forever! It think it's only supposed to be like 1 hour and it felt like we were in the air forever and a day. I seriously took two naps during this flight! I think they were circling or something. I don't know. Those weirdos... So like the second time I woke up, I got up to pee and the flight attendant (there was only one because this plane was sooo soo tiny) literally yelled at me!!! She goes (now make this sound really nasally, "The Nanny" style) "We are landing!!! You need to be in your seat!!" Dang... good thing I was able to hold it the next hour that we were circling and taxi-ing and god knows what.

:)

Anyway. Where was I? I was a little bit uncomfortable in the seats because the planes were the oldest, dinkiest things ever. I should mention the airline... but I won't because I'm sure soon enough they'll all be like that with all the problems they're having. I always wonder how normal sized people feel in these planes. I'm very short and I kept hitting my head and knocking my knees so I wonder how someone 6' feels...

So I'm out here on vacation having a little downtime. Trying to regroup so that I can tackle these next couple of months I have until the baby is born. I, of course, want everything to be perfect! So I'm gonna work my fanny off to whip my family into shape! I'm outta town for 4 days and dear bf has been skipping meals and staying up all night! I shoulda cooked some things for him to warm up before I left... that weenie! He knows how to cook! Better than me!

Feeling Good!!

So I'm almost halfway through! I'm feeling huge today... I just ate lunch, and I think I ate too much. I'm wearing one of my pre-pregnancy skirts. It's a little tight so I think that it's going to have to go to the back of the closet! It fit this morning!!

I'm starting to show a lot. People are asking me if I'm pregnant and when I'm due and all that jazz... It's kinda fun. It still kinda feels weird to me that I'm pregnant, but I'm getting really excited. We won't know the sex until the ultrasound on Aug. 9th, but we've already started buying just a few little things. I bought some onesies with my mother when I was out visiting her. And the other night we bought some itty bitty socks. I can't wait until we get a dresser and a crib so I'll have a place to put stuff! I really can't wait until we find out if it's a boy or a girl. My boyfriend said that I should really stop calling it a boy or a girl until we find out for sure. I don't know. I'm still kinda sure that my initial hunch is right. We'll see.

I was thinking back on the beginning of everything. I never really wrote too much about it because I was sooo in shock that *I* was pregnant! I'm still in shock kinda but it's cool being pregnant. She moves (oops...) The baby moves so much now. Yesterday I swear it was awake for like 6 hours last night kicking and such. I said, "baby, don't think you're going to be up this late when you're born!!" It better take after me and like sleep. Enyway, back to the beginning of everything. I actually had peed on so many sticks month after month that I was not ever expecting a positive. Then one day in April the day that AF was due, I peed on a dollar tree one on a lark. I figured, hey, at only $1, I could do this every day! As I sat down to go, (warning to sensitive folks this gets graphic) one tiny drop of blood dripped into the water. I was like, oh well, here we go again. I peed on the stick anyway and stuck on a pantiliner. A very very faint line appeared right away and I shoved it in the cabinet...

I really have to go back to work so this story is "to be continued".

So I hid the test in the cabinet and I kept looking at it and looking at it... I had been surfing the web and found that most places said that if there is any line at all, no matter how faint, that means it's probably positive. So a couple of hours later I finally decided to show dear bf. I looked at him incredulously, and said "I think it's a positive... but I don't know!!" It can't be; can it? Since I had let it sit for so long, the line got darker so we both doubted it. But there was no more spotting for the rest of the weekend. I decided to go in to get tested officially the Tuesday afterwards- the first test I took was on a Friday. I still doubted it because so many times before I was late and then what do you know... Then we found out for sure and I still doubted it until (despite the nausea, gas, headaches, hiccups, sore bbs, frequent urination, lack of AF) I heard the heartbeat weeks later. And to be honest, it's just now becoming really real because I'm getting so big! And all of the kicking- I can see it on the outside now, so that's really cool. I just can't wait to see the ultrasound to make sure it's okay and find out what it is!

Sorry for TMI (if any of it was), I just want to remember all of this stuff!

2006-08-01 (19 weeks)

Kickin' Like Crazy...

So this baby seems to be in motion a lot! I hope it's moving around a ton when we have the ultrasound on the 9th. It just gave me a huge kick- the biggest one yet! I can definitely feel them on the outside now. The baby seems to move the most right around 11 pm when mommy and daddy are starting to go to sleep!

I got a nice body pillow to sleep with. It's wonderful. I don't think it's a real body pillow but rather a king size pillow- but um, it seems to be as long as my body!! Last night the whole family, including Zimmy the cat, slept in our room. It was real cozy. Although Zimmy and my future stepson crashed out on the floor. There's just no room for all of us in the bed now with me, my big-ole belly, my body pillow and my dear bf...

Anyway, I gotta get back to work!!

2006-08-03 (19 weeks)

Leg Cramps???

Okay, I've been having leg cramps all day today! The other night I woke up with a charlie horse in my calf and the cramps today are in the same leg. I've got cramps in my thigh and in my calf and now I feel one in my foot.

So what do I do??? eek!! And I'm feeling kind of dizzy. I wonder if one has to do with the other? I may have forgotten to take my vitamin today. That may be why. I hate when I forget if I forgot or not... Then I'm like, uh, well, if I did take it I shouldn't really have another one but if I didn't take it I should take one... It's all very complicated!! Maybe I should get one of those pill cases with the days of the week on there.

So my sister, who is also expecting and due in December, was supposed to find out yesterday what she was having. I haven't talked to her yet! She better email me or something soon!

My Sister's Having A...

My sister's having a boy! Yay! We talked on the phone last night longer than we have ever talked on the phone, I think. She has no idea what she wants to name him. I'm sure our dad will be happy to get a little boy in the family! It's been a long time since we had a little baby, and this one's going to be a boy!!

So maybe this increase the chances that the little bambino I'm carrying will be a girl?

Okay, I have to get back to work. Man, I don't think I brought enough donuts this morning...

Nothing Much

Nothing much to report, I guess. My belly feels kinda small today so of course I'm freaking out, but I do feel a lot of stretching going on down there. I don't know. The ultrasound is in 2 days. Less than 48 hours, even... So then I will finally know what's in there! I asked dear bf if he would freak out if it had antennae or something like that. I don't know what I'm thinking. I'm almost positive it's not an alien.

But seriously. I wonder if it's really a girl? I don't know. I'm pretty good at predicting. I had a fleeting thought once after conception that it was a boy but ever since the first kick I've been thinking it's a girl. We'll see. My friend who is due in October says that her baby was crossing its legs during the ultrasound so they couldn't tell. I'm starting to think they're pulling one over on us, I mean, can a baby really cross its legs the entire time during the ultrasound?

It's A....

Baby Boy!!

So much for my flawless baby-sex predicting record! hah!! Maybe I'm just right about other people's babies...

A boy. hmph... it's still sinking in. I've never really dealt with a boy baby. He's gonna be a momma's boy, that's for sure. I guess you gotta love boys. They always love their mommies. Even during the teenage years. But they sure are stinky...

I've got to think of a nursery theme. I told my dear bf that I was still decorating it with butterflies. :) I'll have to think of some other cool thing. I guess the under the sea theme or winnie the pooh? Maybe I can find something cute with bugs or lizards. I'm not diggin' the boats and trucks theme... kinda boring. Maybe a beachy thing with lizards and pails. That sounds kinda cute.

He's going to be the cutest, smartest little thing ever!

Dear bf wants to name him Gregory Joseph. Gregory after my dad (and brother) and Joseph after his best friend and his cousin. It's growing on me... I'm so used to yelling out "Greeegooorryyy...." to tick off my brother all these years.

I'll try to get the ultrasound pics on here this evening.

A boy. :)

Ultrasound Pics!!

The ultrasound pics are up!

Doctor Today

Life is busy busy busy. We have to go to the doctor today for the follow-up on the ultrasound. I guess I get to hear the results from the screenings they did for birth defects too. I hope all is well. I need to remind myself to ask the doctor about prenatal classes... There's all kinds of things that I could pay for, but I'm looking for the free stuff! Maybe I'll take a yoga or swim class that I pay for though.

My dear stepson started school today, so that's pretty exciting- big 1st grade! I don't know what happened last night. He managed to break the free calculator that my mom mailed to him (one of them, I didn't tell him there are more...). Or I think that maybe the battery ran out on it, but he definitely broke it trying to "fix" it after that!! So well, anyway, he's freaking out because he's convinced that he's going to need a calculator for math (1st grade, mind you). T'was quite funny. I told him that he's just gonna have to learn the stuff without a calculator. And so I was so busy with him last night because he's lost his appetite due to the medicine he's on now that I was trying to figure out what to feed him besides McDonald's (ended up giving him subway) that I forgot completely about his dad maybe being hungry when he got home from work. oops...

Ah well, I had other stuff to do! I was feeding the kid and I also had to cut out the flash cards the teacher sent home with us to cut out while trying to convince dear stepson that she wanted specifically for the parents to do this... and filling out papers and all of that stuff, you know.

Anyway. Back to work.

Gaining Weight

So I guess I've gained 8 pounds in the last month for a total of 14 pounds since I've been pregnant. Ugh... I think that is too much so I'm cutting some things out and making sure I get plenty of fruits and vegetables. So, no more pop, donuts, chips. I have to have the occasional french fry since I'm a french fry addict. I think I'll be okay as long as I cut out the pastries. That's one thing I have gone overboard on, I think.

Enough about me!! The baby is doing great so far. He feels huge down there, but I guess 14 ounces is not too big for his age. Especially since he's 3 days older than we thought. The ultrasound said the due date is Dec. 19 instead of the 22nd. They're not going to change it since we were so close. In fact, my original guess was the 21st and they were the ones to say the 22nd! I knew it. I'm still holding out for him to be born on the 22nd since that's the first day of winter but we shall see.

So we were so excited that we went out and spent money on clothes at the consignment shop. We spent almost 70 bucks! But we got some cool stuff. We got a little snow suit! So cute... It's just a plain blue one. So if I see one of those ones that have like the animal ears on it- I'm going to get it too. And we got some cute little outfits and sleepers.

I've been a little blue lately, too. I took the day off yesterday intending to clean the house a little and ended up moping around. It's been really tough adjusting to my new role as a stepmom. The idea of being alone with the kid some days gives me a lot of anxiety since the transition of him moving in with us has been harder than anticipated. I don't know if I can do it all! But anyways. I've been a bit overwhelmed and it's been hard to catch my breath. Some days I just want to sit back and enjoy my increasingly round belly...

And people seriously need to quit commenting on my size! I'm going to freak out! I'm not that stinkin' big, people! I weigh 133 pounds now.

2006-08-17 (21 weeks)

I'm Forgetting Stuff!!

Just so I remember...

So little what's-his-name (I'm not sold on the name his Daddy picked) has been kicking like crazy. You can see it on the outside! Just yesterday while we were trying to light the grill I was sitting back and his dad saw my belly move. He says he's been feeling movement for weeks, but to actually see it like that is a different thing altogether!!

So now that he's moving so much I'm starting to feel a real bond with him... it's cool.

I better go now. It's dinner time!

Perms and Relaxers?

So I hear from many sources that you shouldn't perm or relax your hair during pregnancy. Anyone else hear this?

I'm trying to think of my alternatives here because my hair is getting kinda crazy!! I've mainly just been pulling it back and putting lots of hair gel on it. :)

Definitely Pregnant...

So people come up to me now and ask me when I'm due. I guess it's really obvious that I'm pregnant now! I enjoy being pregnant, everyone is being sooo nice to me. It makes me kind of suspicious the way people are being nice to me... :) It's like "don't open that jar, you're pregnant" "no, you go first, you're pregnant" "here let me carry that for you" "sit down, you're pregnant" I feel like I just want to stay pregnant because I fear what'll happen afterwards! It's like I'm going to jump out of my maternity clothes into some serious work clothes. "You're not pregnant anymore-scrub this floor, cook some food, move this furniture..."

I don't know. Probably irrational!

But the other day at the grocery store I did play the pregnancy card for the first time (other than at home). I was pretty fired up, but I'm not the yelling type so I just had the girl go back to get me some new ricotta cheese. I was at home cooking, so proud of myself because I decided to make something new, stuffed shells... I've got the sauce bubbling, the shells boiling and I cracked open the ricotta cheese. It was sealed and everything. It wasn't even expired- I had just bought it 2 days before and I look inside and there was a ring of mold right in the middle of it. Admittedly, I thought about just spooning the mold out, but I thought, no, there's no telling what's in there that's naked to the eye, ya know. I'm pregnant so I better not take any chances. So I hauled my pregnant butt back up to the grocery store; I was just there buying milk before I started cooking! And so I tell the girl behind the service counter about it and she kinda just gave me a blank look. "Do you want a new one" she says. um... yah, you weirdo... No, I was just going to eat the bad one but I wanted to show you. She says "well, just go get a new one" and I asked her if someone could go get it for me. And she did. What ever happened to customer service?

I didn't mention the pots of boiling food I had to turn off and cover up and the fact that most of the shells were ruined. But it actually ended up turning out okay. There's only 3 of us, so the shells I salvaged fed us for dinner and the boys' lunch the next day.

But anyway. Back to work!

Braxton Hicks

I already started writing this entry but for some reason the page shut off and I lost the entry!! So anyways. I think I've had my first Braxton Hicks contraction. I mean the other night I think one woke me up while I was sleeping. I woke up and my back was hurting until I kept tossing and turning. But this last one... I think it was the real deal. I was just sitting there on the bus and this pain bubbled up like a football-sized gas bubble. It made my toes curl. I don't think I changed my facial expression any but my foot was shakin'. Well, anyway, it bubbled up and just hurt for I don't know how long, but then it just went away. Maybe it was just the baby trying to do something. I don't know.

I'm starting to feel achy. My back aches at work and my legs cramp up. I enjoy being pregnant still though. Mostly when I'm laying back and rubbing my belly. Speaking of which- is it obscene to rub your belly in public? Some people look at me weird when I do it. I mean, everyone else reaches out and touches my belly... I should be able to too!

Created Registry!!

Okay, I finally created the registry. Actually I did 3! I started at Target and then went to Babies R Us and then to Walmart. There's not much at Walmart because I couldn't find anything there... Anyway. All three are online and in the store.

To my family and friends- if you'd like to buy me something that I put on the Target registry and you find it cheaper somewhere else, just let me know and I'll take if off. I just need stuff. I'm not partial to any brand or anything!

<u>Baby Hiccups???</u>

Anyone else's baby have hiccups all the time? Seems like all the kicking has been replaced with hic, hic, hic movements... He's got me worried. Again. :)

There is good news though... I haven't gained any weight in the last 2 weeks, so I'm on target for my 25-35 pound weight gain. I guess cutting out the donuts worked or maybe he just had a big growth spurt last month or something. I went to WIC yesterday and they weighed me and had me fill out a chart of what I ate in the past 24 hours. I guess I'm doing a good job! She did say to make sure I ate more veggies and I was actually short on meat servings. But that was Sunday and Sunday was a busy day.

Names...

So, I think that I'm over the original pick for the name. We've still got Joseph, but we need a name to go with it!! Nothing is working out yet.

Decided on a Name! (I Think...)

So last night we finally agreed on Elijah Joseph. I really love that name! Let's see if I keep it! :)

I got some tummy pics back and I will be posting them ASAP. I was happy to see that I am not nearly as huge as I feel. :) Although people still comment on how huge I am. They must not realize how big a ninth-month belly is... I'm no where near that, I think! Oh well, I love my belly no matter what people say! It's awesome to have a baby in there. And his kicking was back to normal yesterday. I'm hoping for another good day of kicking today. I realize that I'm only 24 weeks along so the kicking is not really that regular, but I still freak out when I notice differences, you know?

So as far as the prenatal classes... I'm bummed out! There is a (seemingly) awesome prenatal/postnatal swim class at the YMCA by me, but it's Tuesdays during the day! Maybe I'll take it after I give birth? I don't know. I kinda want to take it now! The YMCA near me is really nice, too. I might have to go to another one, but I think another nice one is all the way up north.

And then the birthing classes that I need to take, well, the free ones are in a not-so-desirable neighborhood at night... eek... I'm not going. I don't think anyone would hurt me or anything, but just seeing people hanging out at night looking all seedy-looking... Anyway. I think I'd rather pay for something but I don't know what dear bf is going to say about that. There's a ton of hospitals in this town and I'm sure one of them offers something... The hospital where my baby will be born offers classes for $175. I should probably go there since it ends with a tour of labor and delivery. And also going there like 8 weeks in a row will help me remember where the place is, you know.

I should be working now. :)

Belly Pics!!

Belly pics are up!!

Olive Garden for Shower?

My future MIL and SIL are trying to talk me out of having the baby shower at the Olive Garden. They want me to have it at my apartment's clubhouse so that we can play games and decorate. I think we can still play the games at the Olive Garden, and I'm okay with not having decorations. I don't want to do the clubhouse because we'd have to provide the food, and I'm not too creative with party food. MIL suggested a meat and cheese tray but I don't know. I have some friends that would have to drive up 45 min, and I don't think they'd do it for a meat and cheese tray. Not to mention that me and my other prego friend should not be eating lunch meat!

Any suggestions??? Like, ideas for food or perhaps another restaurant that would be more intimate or conducive for a shower?

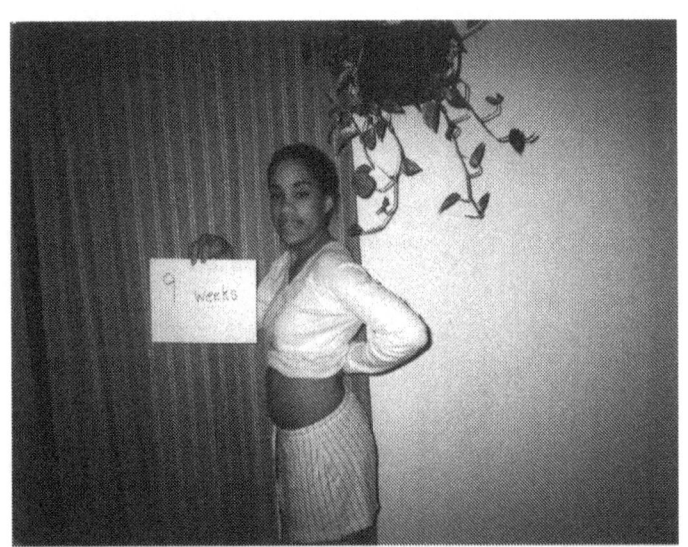

9 weeks

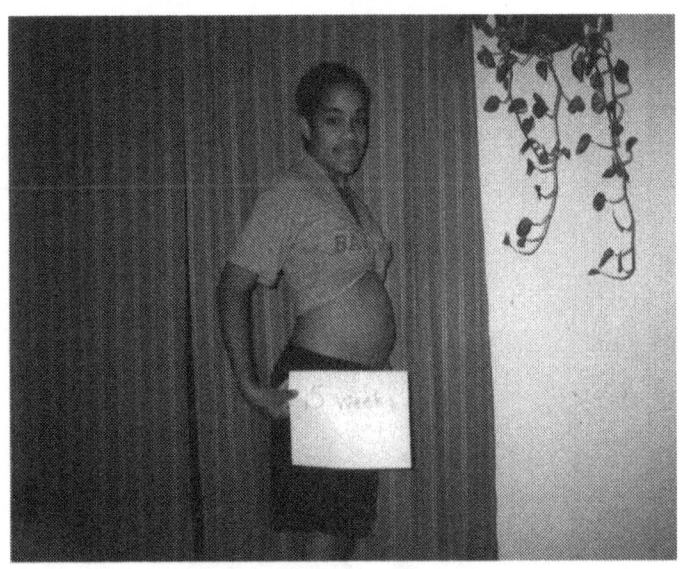

15 weeks

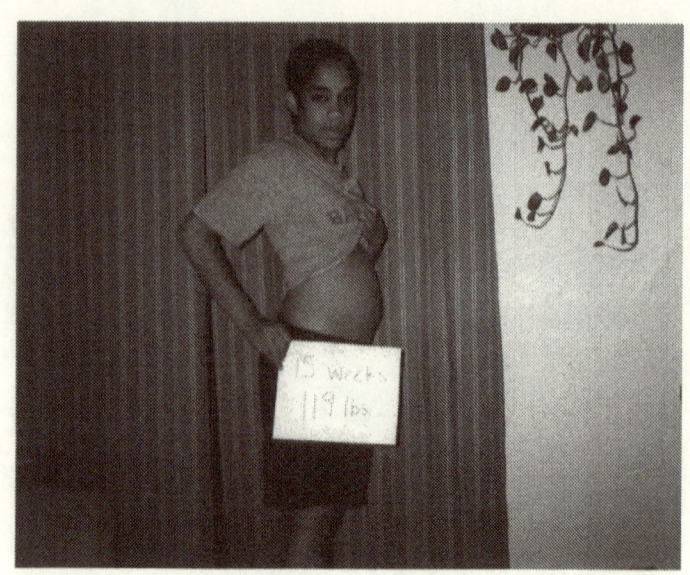

15 weeks (119 lbs.)

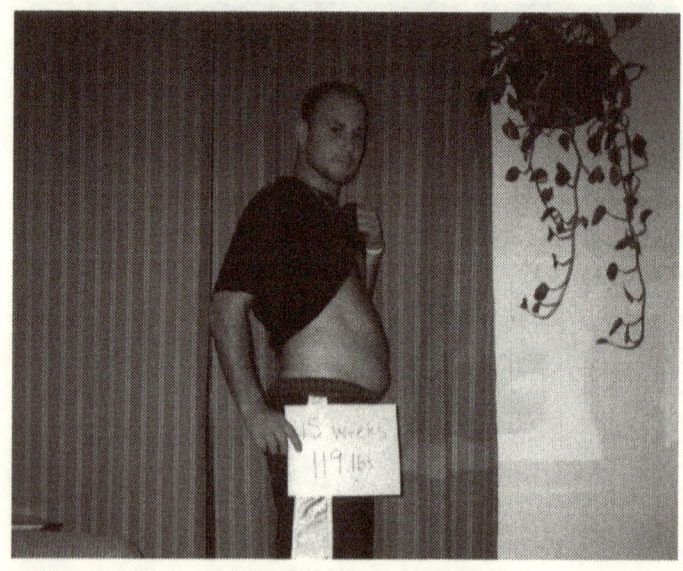

Daddy, 15 weeks

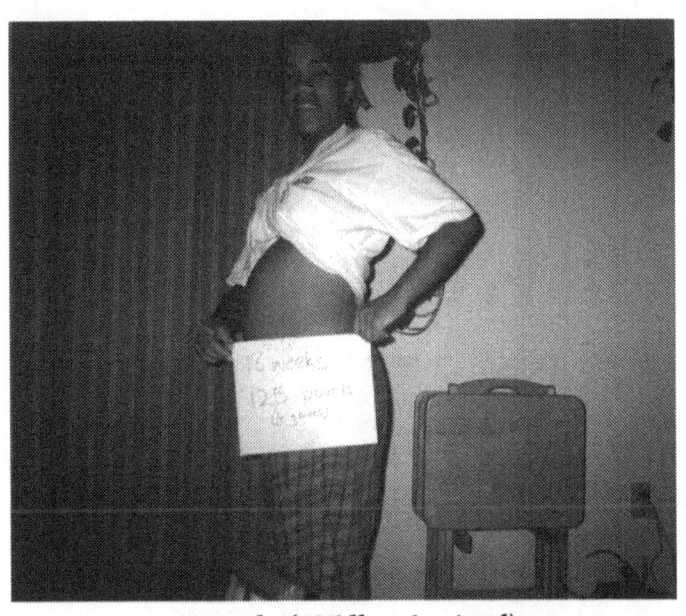

18 weeks (125 lbs., 6 gained)

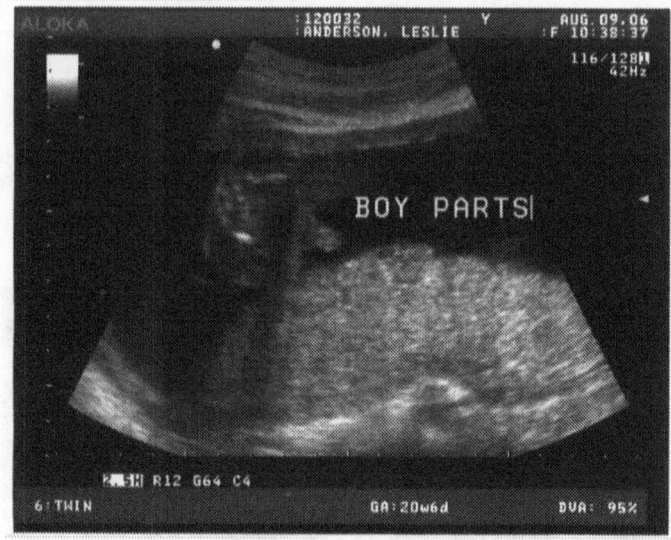

Boy parts

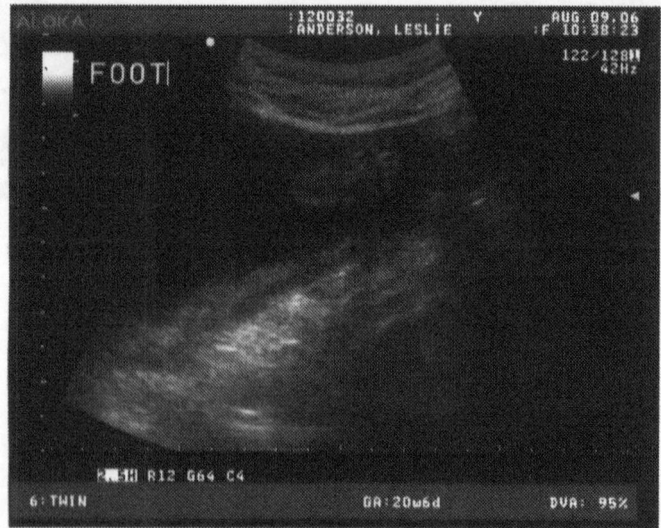

Baby foot

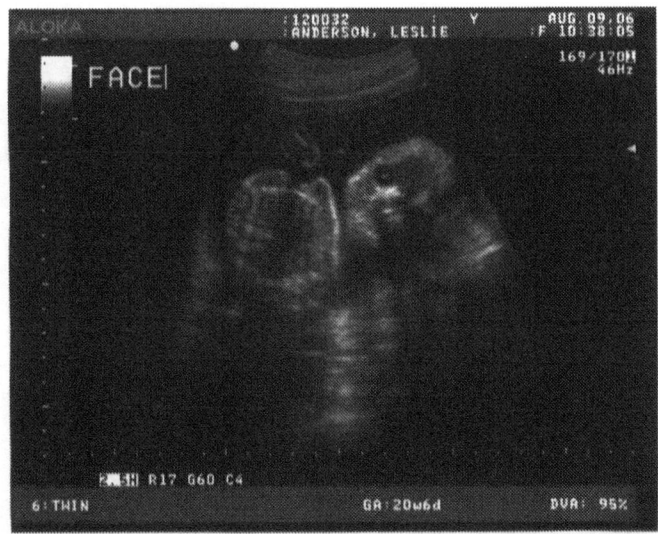

Baby face

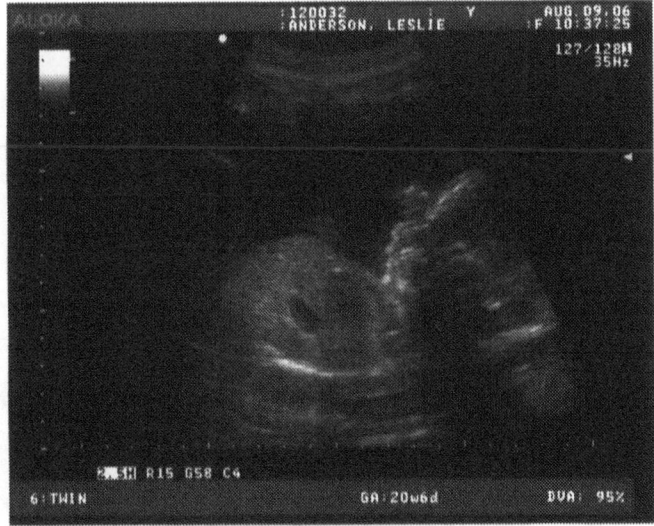

Baby profile

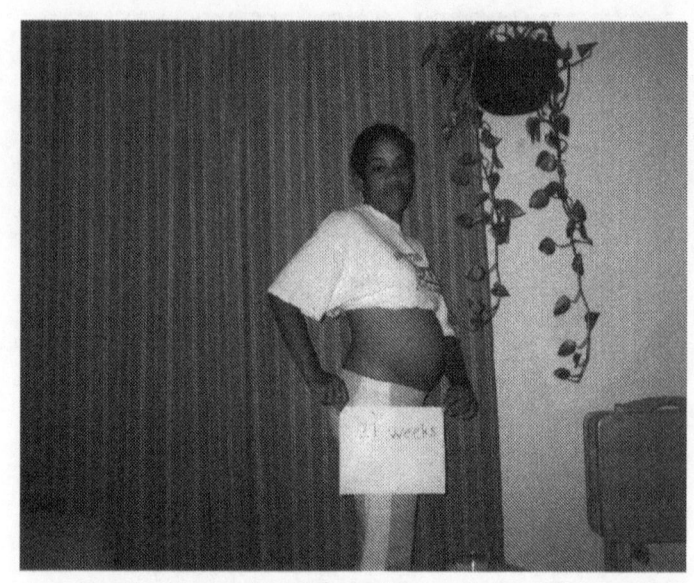

21 weeks

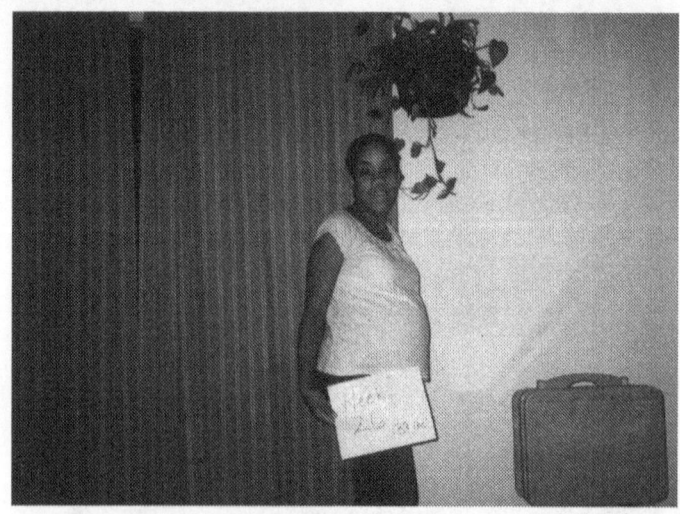

26 weeks (139 lbs.)

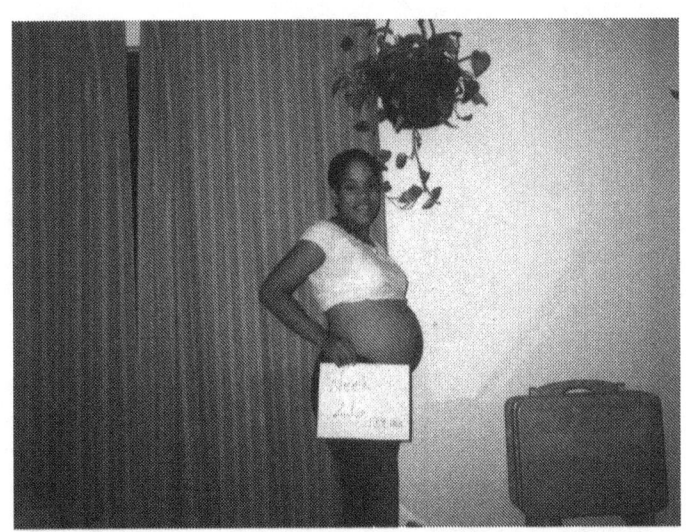

26 weeks (139 lbs.)

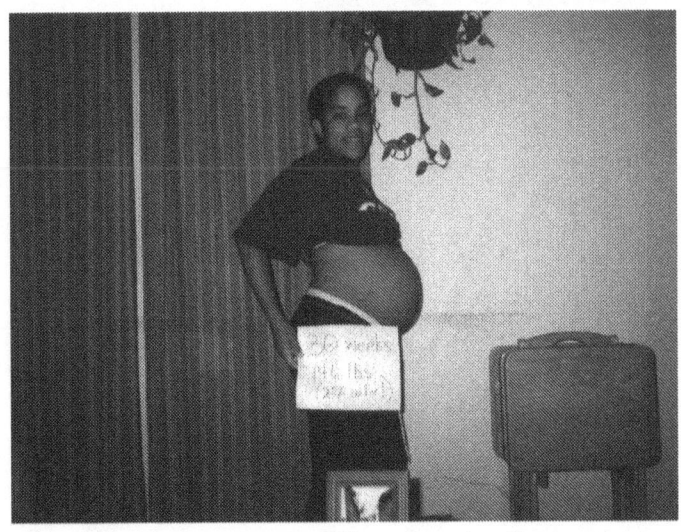

30 weeks (146 lbs., 27 gained)

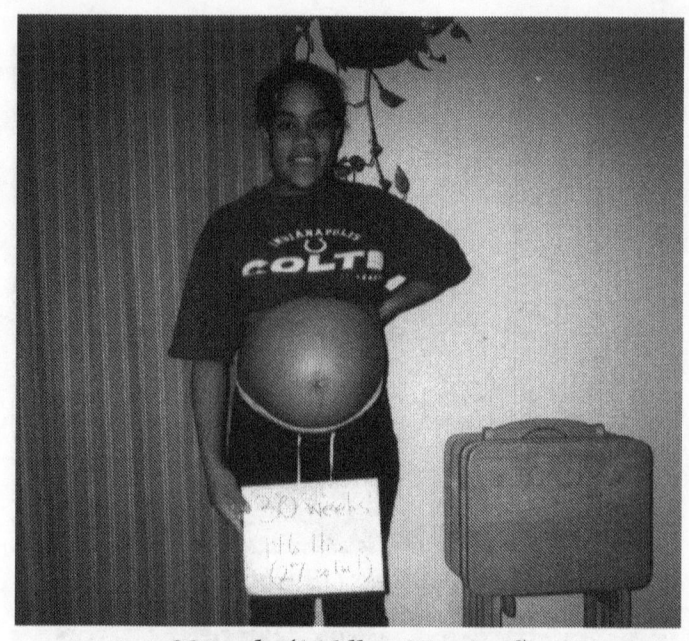

30 weeks (146 lbs., 27 gained)

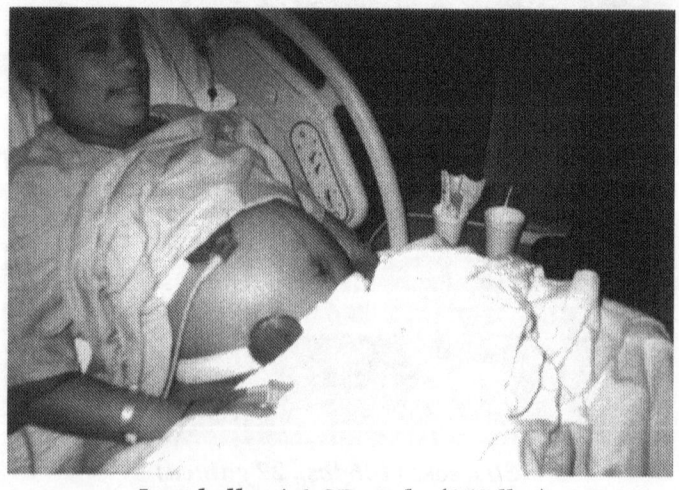

Last belly pic! 37 weeks (153 lbs.)

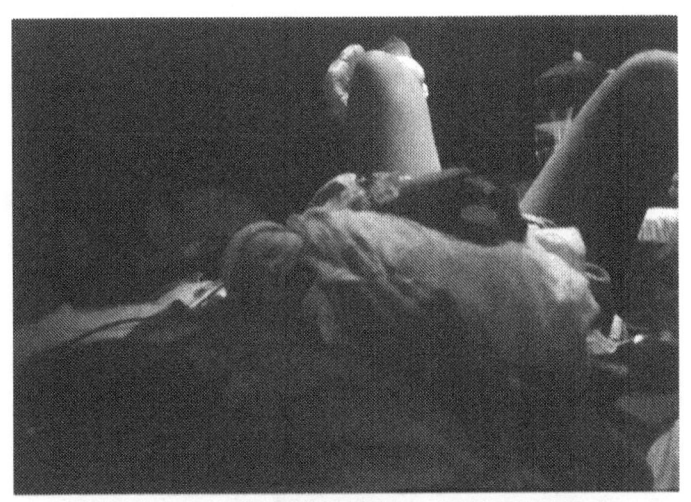

Mommy and Elijah shortly after delivery

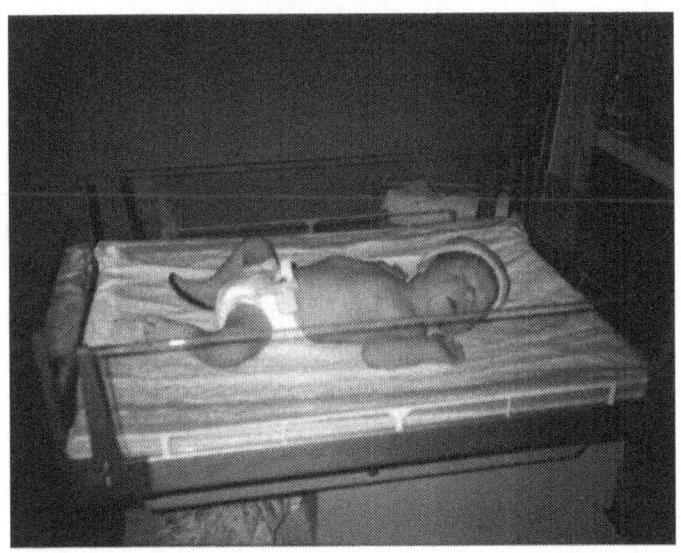

Elijah Joseph Bose (forceps bruise on forehead)

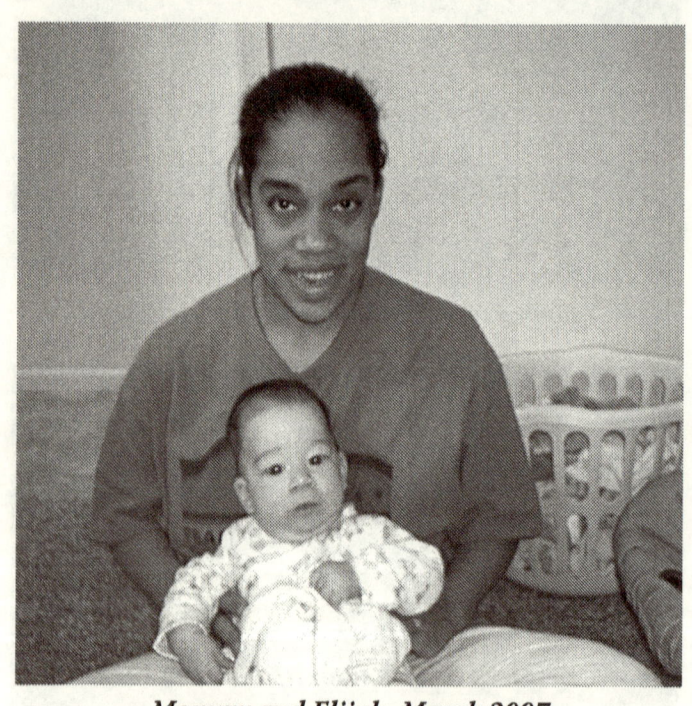

Mommy and Elijah, March 2007

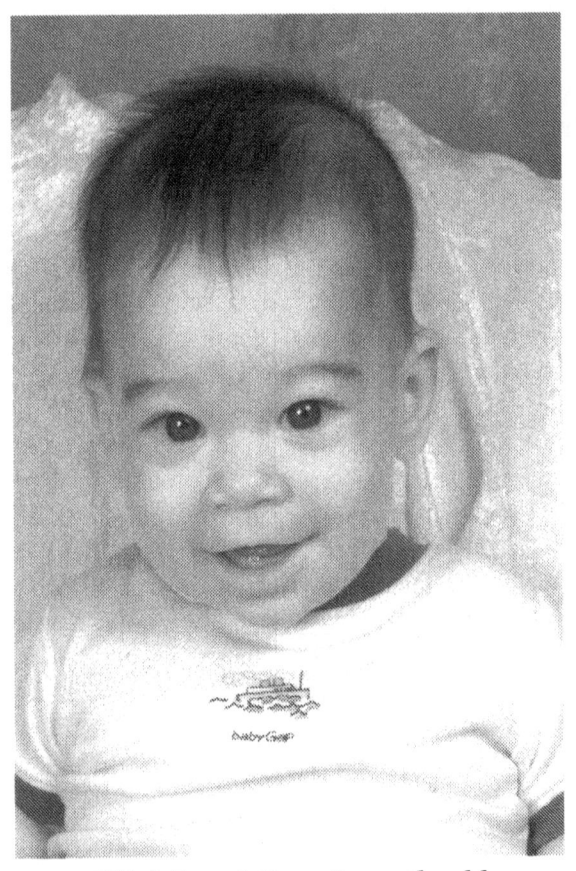

Elijah Joseph Bose, 6 months old

Swollen Feet

My feet are swollen! It must be really bad because dear bf can tell! My little feet are fat anyway, so for a long time no one else could tell that they were bigger than normal.

I haven't really written a lot about anything. Stuff has been happening so quickly, I can't tell up from down! I need to take some new belly pics. It's already the end of week 25, and I haven't taken a pic since week 21 I think. Wow! The time is flying by. All of us are bringing jackets with us in the morning because the weather is already cooling off. Summer zoomed by really fast. I think it goes faster now that I'm older. My birthday is coming up soon and then it will be fall! Yowsa...

Anyway, this is supposed to be about the pregnancy and stuff. We're starting to get things together. I put the registry together and people are already buying stuff. It is so very exciting. :) I think I want to be pregnant forever! No wonder people get depressed after the birth... I'm kind of nervous about that actually. It's like you're the princess during pregnancy- then after pregnancy, who knows- lowly servant? I don't know. I suppose life is what you make of it. I can't wait to see Elijah. I think after pregnancy I'll be blissful earth mother. :) Hopefully by then I can get step son in line so he's a helper. And crazy bf? Gotta love 'im...

48

Got the Crib

Okay guys, in case we don't get the invitations out any time soon, the baby shower is going to be Sept. 30th at my apartment clubhouse!!

I haven't done anything today. Oh well, that's what I was told to do by dear bf. I was really tired after breakfast, so he just told me to lay back and relax all day. So that's what I did. :) We took off the entire day tomorrow because it is his birthday, so we're just going to take care of everything tomorrow- grocery shopping and all of that jazz. Maybe I'll make him a cake and dinner. I already bought his present- tickets to a Cubs/Reds game. That should be fun, it's on the 25th.

Man... I don't know why I'm so tired!! Maybe the honeymoon 2nd trimester is coming to a close? I think I'm still pretty fit but I get worn out easier. I want to take a prenatal water aerobics class- has anyone else done that? There is one that starts this week, so that would be 8 weeks during my 6th and 7th month. The one after that starts in November, so that would be during my 8th and 9th month; ending like a week before my due date. I wonder if that would be too taxing on me? I don't know! Maybe that would be better because I'll still be all fit and ready for labor? Maybe that would bring on early labor though??? I don't know. It's not like it's strenuous or anything. I need to ask the doctor when I go tomorrow. Decisions, decisions. Plus I still need to take labor preparation classes...

enywoo... I wonder why I have this urge to take on like a million things??? Oh well. I just want to make everything perfect.

The crib- :) So dear bf's dad was nice enough to help us pay off the crib! So we've got that taken care of. I didn't think that we'd have that paid off yet, so that's awesome. I went ahead and put a changing table/dresser on layaway. I'm putting the pic of the crib and changing table/dresser up in the photo album. I don't want the armoire that's in the picture. I don't think we'll need it. Who knows, I guess. But with his dresser and crib, the kid already has more bedroom furniture than me!

But I'd better quit my rambling. I'm off to create more lists of stuff to do!

2006-09-11 (25 weeks)

Doctor Appointment Today

I went to the doctor today and the baby is still doing great! Man, I love him so much!! He's so big now she didn't have to hunt for him to hear the heartbeat. He had his head down and his butt up for the appointment, but I think he flips around a ton.

Oh. I gained 5.5 more pounds. Eek... So now I'm up to 139! 139... jeez oh peez! That's 20 pounds overall. I still don't think I'm huge, but oh well. 20 pounds. I think that's all the baby. :) Hah! But nonetheless, eek... She recommended that if I wanted to take the prenatal water fitness class, I should take the one that starts on Saturday. That means I have to run out and get a suit. She said that I probably won't want to start anything in my 8th and 9th month. That makes sense. But maybe after this 8 weeks ends, I'll either take another class or just do the exercises on my own?

I'm chomping at the bit right now because I have a big UPS package coming from my mom. I asked UPS if they could come after 2. Hopefully they don't come too late. I know that sometimes they can deliver at night.

I better go!

Who Bought The...

Okay, I'm guilty... I've been looking at the registries to see what stuff is getting purchased. But so anyway, somebody bought a Boppy and I have no idea who it was. I wonder if it was someone for me or maybe someone printed up the wrong registry? Who knows.

I bought myself more maternity clothes- I spent like $80. I think I'm finished. I should have enough to make it through. I probably have to buy at least one pair of shoes though. I think my feet are getting bigger... But I bought a cool pair of jeans, a black skirt, some khaki pants and a shirt. Not a lot for $80 bucks, but I really needed to get some stuff and my priority was finding stuff that fit. I actually went into Goodwill and tried to find some things before I went to the mall. I had to search through two racks of things- they had the plus sizes mixed in with the maternity stuff... Then I found like 6 things to try on and out of that, only 2 shirts were keepers. Upon closer inspection, one of the shirts had a stain on it. It wasn't really noticeable, but I prefer not pay ($3 or no $3) for someone else's stains. I mean, I'm not a picky person and sometimes I wear my own stains for a while before I throw something out, but you know. Anyway. So I just left that shirt and the other one there and headed off to

Motherhood. And they didn't really have a lot of stuff there! But I hunted around and found what I found and hopefully it'll last through my due date.

Swollen Legs

Okay, I'm freaking out again. My swollen ankles have now turned into swollen legs! I had it yesterday and it went away over night, but now it's back again today. I've been trying not to cross my legs and trying to drink plenty of water. We'll see if it gets as bad as it was last night. At first I was freaking out thinking that maybe I was just getting that fat... Then I realized that my legs were floating in the tub more than usual.

I guess I should have given up crossing my legs earlier than now, but I didn't see anything wrong with it until now. I called the doctor just as a precaution, but I haven't heard anything from them yet. Hopefully they'll leave me a message this afternoon. I was just in there on Monday and I'm pretty sure my blood pressure and everything was okay. I forgot to mention the puffy ankles, and now I have puffy legs. And I'm wearing a skirt today.

If it ain't one thing, it's another!

Pre-natal Water Fitness Class

So I drove all the way up to the YMCA on the other side of town to begin my class on Saturday (after a huge drag 'em out fight with my future stepson to get him out of bed) and there was nobody there!! They cancelled the class due to low enrollment and did not bother to call me. Bums. I was more disappointed than mad though. I want to take my darned pre-natal water fitness class!! Ugh.

There has got to be something in this town that I can do! I think I've seen yoga classes, but I'm not into yoga, really. I guess the point would be to meet other pregos anyway. My fantasy pregnancy is not going as planned!! I don't really have too many expectations, I just want to be fit & meet some friends I guess. Ugh.

Elijah is moving around in there. He's probably telling mommy to go get something to eat! It's lunchtime!

2006-09-20 (26 weeks)

Shooting Leg Pains

So yesterday I was talking to my co-worker about my incessant hiccups. I've had hiccups since I found out I was pregnant!! I swear. I said that I'm so bored with the hiccups. I'm ready for a new symptom. So. What happens??? I end up with shooting leg pains. Lovely!

The girls in the office who've been pregnant (otherwise known as my source of all sorts of labor horror stories...) tell me that this whole leg cramp, leg swelling, shooting leg pain, etc. thing is normal. Argh! I guess that's what happens when you have a big old 20 pound belly strapped onto you. I swear that's the only place I've gained weight, so all 20 have to be right there in front. I may have put on a few pounds in my rear end, but so far there's no gain in my face or boobs or anything.

This shooting leg pain thing seems to happen when I'm sitting still or standing still mostly, so I'm thinking that it felt so bad after work yesterday because I was standing at the bus stop for a while and then sitting on the bus for a while. It's not too bad during worktime (yet!) because I have to get up a lot and run to the printer. If I keep moving, it's more of a dull achy feeling whereas when I sit or stand still for too long, the shooting pain happens. I think I'm too small to have a child. He can't possibly have any room in there and there's no way that I can possibly get any bigger. I'm gonna end up in one of those pregnancy sling things. This morning I was thinking- what if I have to stop working soon. What the heck would I do? Anyway. Positive thoughts... I think I just need to get moving and exercise a little bit more. (by more I mean any at all...) My body needs to get used to all of this weight up front.

2006-09-21 (26 weeks)

Stayed Home (Again) Today

So last night dear bf was checking out my legs around 10 o'clock and they were the size of watermelons!! They were huge. So he started freaking out and telling me I had to go to the doctor and not to even go to work today. So I didn't. I went there and they weren't even going to see me until I said that I was feeling tingling in my fingers too. The first nurse seemed like she freaked out when she heard that. But I guess that it just from typing so much! I need to get a gel pad for my keyboard at work and the one at home. I'm sure I could get them to buy that for me at work- or maybe the temp agency will.

I gotta eat something. I'll write more later.

Big 2-9

So I've been the teensiest bit depressed as my birthday approaches. I'm going to be 29 tomorrow. It kinda makes me nauseous to think about it. Elijah's only going to know his mommy as an old lady.

Oh yeah, I never finished about the doctor yesterday. Everything is fine. I just overdid it working and then spending a few hours at the laundromat. I just always try to squeeze too much in whenever dear bf is off so I have some help with my future stepson. But I need to drink more water and eat less bad food. Last night I think I did alright- I had a nice piece of baked salmon, broccoli and noodle-thingys with a full glass of pineapple juice (with some imaginary coconut rum) and a full glass of water. Needless to say I peed all night, but I think it was all very healthy peeing.

Craziness!!!

So the baby shower is this weekend, and I've been running around like a chicken with its head cut off. Mostly because my mother is coming to town tomorrow! I've been trying to clean up in between working and everything, and it has been crazy!! I actually swept and mopped the kitchen floor this morning at 5:30 after ushering dear bf off to work. I was going to do that last night but my legs were swollen again. I'm going to try to drink a lot of water today, so hopefully they won't be as bad and I'll have more energy. We did some cleaning this weekend, but it's a wreck again! The 6-year-old tornado whirled his way through the bathroom and his bedroom... It's sheer craziness in there!!

But so anyway. I need to relax, do what I can and just relax...

The baby is doing great. Right now he's dancing on my bladder, so I'd better get going. :)

2006-09-28 (27 weeks)

Clean House!

So the apartment is now somewhat presentable. I still need to vacuum the little one's room, and our room... I think I'm just going to close the door! Hah! j/k. Our room is not that bad, it just has too many clothes in there. And I've got like 50 library books in there- not helping things!! The clothes are not mine though. I've only got like 6 different prego outfits- and then a bunch of stretch/sweatpants and T-shirts. I get a lot of flack for my shoe collection though. Bf has noooo idea. None! I only have like 20 pair. In my younger days I had twice as many. That whole closet would have been taken up with just my shoes. Besides, half the ones I have now I cannot wear because they're heels or otherwise too dangerous or too uncomfortable to wear during pregnancy. So anyways.

The baby doesn't seem to be up to too much. He does seem like he is huge in there. My mother sent him more stuff via UPS. She wants to be called Nana, she says. We'll see how that works out for her. She's on her way here, so I'm pretty sure she'll be at the apartment when I get off of work. She says it's a nine-hour drive from her house. I'm thinkin' it's supposed to be more like 11!! So but anyway, this time she sent hats and booties and the baby swing that I really wanted. It's a cute little one that should fit right into our living room.

As far as the pregnancy goes, I continue to feel bigger and bigger. I need to exercise more because I'm getting really stiff at times. I feel like an apple dumpling- short and round. It's good though. I can't imagine not being pregnant- to have my normal body back and baby outside of it seems unreal. It feels like I've been pregnant for at least half my life.

So after this crazy week, I'm going to see about exercise. I think I'm just going to go to the pool and swim. I'm sure every little bit of exercise will benefit me a lot in terms of flexibility and fitness.

getting back to work...

2006-10-02 (28 weeks)

Emily's Baby's Here!

So just like that, my friend Emily had her baby. Just last week I was at her baby shower and she looked fine! Then I guess pre-labor started around Thursday with a bad backache. They went into the doctor and he gave her some pain reliever and sent her home. I think she said he checked her and she was already dialated 2-3 cm. He told her just to stay close to home, but he couldn't tell her whether it would be the next day or the next week! Saturday she stopped by my baby shower for a few minutes. She really looked different, like it was "go" time. I guess she spent the previous few days cleaning and sleeping like in a "nesting" mode. At my shower I took one last pic of the two of us, belly to belly. Then yesterday (Sunday) she calls me in the evening and said that she had the baby that afternoon!! Just like that. She was a prego and now she's a mommy! Incredible. I guess I was thinking that I'd be walking around with this baby in my belly forever, you know. Eventually they do come out and it's a real, live little human. Amazing.

2006-10-09 (29 weeks)

Catching Up...

I'm going to go ahead and try to write a little bit while I am semi-motivated to do so. I've been so busy just running around and crap. I can't imagine what it's going to be like when the little one gets here! So... I had the baby shower a week ago on Sept. 30th. I had fun! I don't know if anyone else did, but that's all good I guess. Baby showers aren't supposed to be rip-roarin' fun, ya know. MIL and SIL did a great job with the decorations and everything. They kept asking me what I liked and I didn't really give them much to go on. My only concern was the food... :) Then I ended up eating McDonald's right before the thing started because I was getting so cranky. But it lasted about 2 hours and most of the friends that I invited showed up, so that was cool.

Cranky is the name of my game right now, I guess! I get so peeved when things don't go perfectly. I need to let things go... or the people around me need to get it together!! Yesterday I was cranky because dear bf was lolly-gagging around all day and didn't get home until 8 or 9. So I was wondering when the perfect time would be to start dinner. Once he got home, he lolly-gagged around (well, he was working on the house...) until like 11 or 12! So we all got into bed entirely too late considering we wake up at like 5 am.

Breathe... in through the nose, out through the mouth...

We took our childbirthing class on Friday and Saturday. That was pretty interesting. They kept us all day on Saturday and boy could that woman talk! :) She talked for like 2 hour stretches, which I think was a little bit much. I mean, I'm used to lectures, but dear bf was Mr. Wiggleworm for the whole afternoon. It was all very interesting to me. I learned a few new techniques for dealing with back pain, so that was cool. I still wish I could take some sort of prenatal exercise class or something to better prepare my body. Oh, such is life. Maybe the next pregnancy will be perfecter.

Plus, dear bf has done this before, so it's not like he was hanging on every word like I was. I've read so many books and websites and stuff, but I still soak up every bit of info I hear. She did have me thinking that I could do it all natural though! Hm... I think my friend Emily only had to take the Nubain, but she exercised her whole pregnancy. (Which I have not...) So she was probably pretty fit. hm... Why would I do it all natural? I don't know. Why does anyone do anything I guess. I mean, I don't want to be so doped up that I don't know what's going on, but I don't want to be so blind with pain that I don't know what's going on. I guess if I start training my body now and working with my "birthing partner" now... My only real goal is to make it to 5 cm and see where I am. And of course all of this is conjecture... I can hear the ones who've done this before laughing at me in my ignorance. Ah well.

I have to go eat lunch! Hungry hungry...

Glucose Test

I had my weigh-in yesterday. 146 pounds, for a total of 27 pounds gained! Goodness gracious... oh me oh my.

Anyway. We'll just focus on good eating and exercise and let the numbers figure themselves out.

The glucose test was not bad at all. The orange drink wasn't too bad, it left a funny aftertaste, but it wasn't anything I couldn't handle. I talked to the nurse midwife and hung around the office for an hour then they took tons of blood. One thing of blood was for some antibody test since I'm Rh negative. I guess they don't automatically give you the shot of rhogam (I think that's how you spell it) if there is a chance that your body may already have the antibodies because it'll just make you have even more antibodies. So, well, anyway... I shouldn't have the antibodies because I've never been pregnant (before now) but you never know. IF I do have the antibodies already and they are increasing, she said something about having to induce labor before the count gets too high. That got dear bf's ears all perked up!! But I think I'm fine and I'll go in there in two weeks and take the rhogam shot. It's strange how all of this works... So delicate is this process, huh? I think everything is great so far despite my disappointments about not having the "perfect pregnancy" (stress-free, fit & having perfect eating). I guess I could start piping in classical music and reading poetry nightly. :) Tonight, that might actually work because dear bf has the day off... We'll see.

I'm starting to go to the doc every two weeks now!!

More Doctor Stuff

I'm trying to remember exactly everything she said... I know that she said to try to cut carbs! Like refined ones- white bread, white rice, potatoes, pasta. I guess they contribute to the bloaty feeling too. Also, I need to try to walk around more at work. I'm not constantly at my desk, but I guess I need to get up for longer periods of time. So at my break I need to go for a walk instead of do this!! At lunchtime I got my butt moving by going downstairs to the cafe (to get a salad to go with my soup for lunch). Last night, we went for a short but brisk walk- the beginning of nightly walks. I think I'll go right after work whenever dear bf is working.

Everything is measuring great, and I'm right on track. So for the people that think I'm huge and going to pop tomorrow, you're wrong. :) She doesn't even think the baby will end up being very big- maybe 6 or 7 pounds. Well, baby, that's all mommy has room for anyway! But we'll see. They're never right about the whole weight prediction thing.

I'm so tired right now! I can't wait to see my bed, actually. :) After my walk, of course. I just feel so guilty because dear bf is so social, he just wants to chit chat and hang out all night. I just want to cuddle up with Zimmy the cat and take a nice nap!

Little Bit Anemic

So my doctor office managed to freak me out over the weekend! One of the nurses called my house while I was at work on Friday and left a message to call into the office. Of course I didn't get the message until like Saturday or something. So I got to imagine all the reasons why they could possibly need me to call all day Saturday and all day Sunday. I thought maybe they were going to tell me that we were going to have this baby this week! But everything is fine with my labs except I turned up a little bit anemic. Probably because I forget to take my vitamins sometimes... Now I have to take an iron supplement. That should make pooping even more fun than it is now.

10 more weeks to go! And I still feel great most of the time. Except for at the end of the day. I just want to go to sleep! Poor bf, we don't get much time together any more. I've been going into the bedroom at 10 pm, and I'm knocked out by 10:30. I mean, he used to wake me up all the time turning on lights and fumbling around and stuff. Now, i'm oblivious to it. Apparently the other night he had the light on and was watching the baby move around with his little hands... All the while I was snoozing! And I guess I have starting snoring! That kills me! hah! I'm not really too embarassed by it, you know? Since I don't normally snore! The first thing I thought when dear bf said that was snoring=sleeping. I must be getting some sleep! Even though it feels like I get up a million times during the night to go to the bathroom. They tell you not to drink water after 9pm, but I do anyway. I'm still trying to get my daily water allowance in at that time! Like today, it's already 1pm almost, and I've only had 2 water servings and a serving of tea. And I've only peed once.

So anyway. One of these days I want to write down a list of the things that I love about being pregnant and the things I don't love about being pregnant. I can think of a few things right off hand.

I love the belly! It's cool. Even though I am starting to get some stretch marks. I can tolerate them as long as I don't end up with a deflated basketball-looking belly after the baby is born. In which case, I may just stay pregnant. But it's cool to see Elijah moving inside of me. He seems to be having a ball in there! He's always on the go. And when he finally goes to sleep, his dad wants to talk to him and get him going again!!

I love people being nice to me. I think I've talked about this before. Even living in the city, people are nice! Guys don't hit on me at the bus stop all the freakin' time. It's nice to just sit back and relax and not worry about the riff raff. :)

I don't love people commenting on how huge I am! I'm getting over this since my nurse midwife insists that I'm right on schedule.

I better get back to work. More on this subject later!

2006-10-25 (31 weeks)

Long Time...

I haven't written in a while! Wow... it's already time to go back to the doctor tomorrow.

Life has been hectic, to say the least. Everyone has been sick, except for me, so far. I've just been really tired and resting a lot. I think my body is fighting off the germ assault. After working in daycares and schools so much, I hope I'm finally getting a little immunity to the sniffles. But nonetheless I've been in a daze since Monday. I'm feeling a little better physically, but mentally I think I'm going coo-coo (how do you spell that? hm...).

Today should be an okay day. Dear bf says that he's getting off of work early today. As long as early is before 7, that is cool with me. That means I don't have to handle all the housework (including dear future stepson) without him.

But last night, my mind was just going nuts. I wasn't thinking about anything in particular. It was just one of those nights when I think, dang, I could use a glass of wine. I didn't have the wine, in case anyone is wondering. But this morning I bought a dark chocolate bar that I'm getting ready to eat after I finish my lunch, so maybe I can sit back and relax with that.

Everything is fine, I should just be able to relax. I just get so uptight when I look at my desk at home and I see all the thank you notes that need to get written out, all the bills that need to be sorted out and filed away, all the baby info and coupons that I need to read and take care of...

So anyway. That's what I've been up to! Elijah has been busy all this time getting bigger and moving around more and more. I really think he's huge now. I think he's taking up some of the space where my bladder needs to go because my capacity has gone down a little bit this week! And the belly is getting bigger too! I have quite a few stretch marks now. That's kinda depressing! I've been using the stretch mark lotion religiously, so I hope it'll help somewhat. It just looks like skin shouldn't do that, you know? Like it's hurting it or something. But Elijah seems to be having a good time still. Although he seems to be gettin a little crowded. Sometimes he'll stretch out with all his little strength and makes my stomach stretch to the max. Right now I don't know what he's doing. Seems like he's stretching down towards my bladder.

But this week I have definitely noticed less capacity and more frequency in my urination (if anyone wanted to know that). It's definitely one of the not-so-great things about pregnancy. It seems like every time I stand up I need to pee. And by the time I get home after riding the bus, I feel like I'm going to pee my pants from holding it!

What else? There's just so much! This past weekend I started on my baby scrapbook! Scrapbooking is so much fun and such an overwhelming hobby! Perfect hobby for me to choose, right? Hah! I just want to put together some good memories. I'm not trying to win the scrapbooking prize of the year or anything. So I went up to my friend Stephanie's and we had a "scrap" with some of our friends. It was really fun. Then later on, dear bf, future stepson and I went down to my old hometown and hung out with my friend Syana. That was fun. We went to the mall and I bought two more shirts. I saw some cute courderouys (eek... that's a hard one to spell) at the maternity store, but I debated whether to buy them or not! I'm only going to be pregnant for 2 more months. Heck, less than two more months!! But I had to buy the shirts because the summer shirts I had are not cutting it. I bought mediums, because I'm starting to hang out of the smalls!!

But now I have to eat my chocolate and get back to work. Here's hopin' the chocolate chemicals do their business on my brain...

Anxious!!

We're ready for Halloween. Dear stepson has his costume ready- he's some kind of ghouly-demon thing. We wanted him to be something cutesy, but oh well. He's gonna scare people with his fake axe thing. But hurry up, Halloween!! Let's get it over with! Onto Christmas!!

I used to think it was obnoxious to see the Christmas decorations up by the Halloween candy in the store, even as recently as last year. But this year! I'm soooo excited for Christmas to be here I want to decorate the house right now! I won't do that because it'll be boring to look at the decorations for the next 2 months (less than two months!!!) But I want everything to be ready for baby's first Christmas! I can see us now, opening a million gifts for little Elijah and he won't know what the heck is going on...

So 8 weeks left. Can you believe it??? that's until my due date, and I am almost positive that he'll be here before then. Man, I think he's ready now! I can't believe there is a baby coming. It's incredible and mind-blowing. But 8 more weeks! To get everything ready? That's amazing. We'll pull it off. I know we will.

I'd better get back to work.

Leaking Water???

I wonder if I'm leaking water? I keep going to the bathroom- little trickles... Oh I don't know what the heck's going on!

I feel like I'm leaking now just sitting here. Maybe I'm just stressed out... In any case, what should I do if I am leaking water? Go to the emergency room?

Hee Hee... No Worries...

Okay, so. I think the baby was just resting on my bladder!! There hasn't been anymore "leaking" since Friday, so I think everything is okay. I'm still convinced this baby is coming sooner rather than later though. Call it mother's intuition. Of course, my intuition led me to believe I was having an Aubrey and not an Elijah... But seriously!! There is no more room down there! Whose idea was it to let a human grow in there for nine months? Just getting bigger and bigger and bigger...

Oh yeah, P.S. We carved pumpkins Friday night. Whew-hew... exciting stuff. Meanwhile, I'm singing Christmas carols in my head... :) At least this weekend we get to do our first round of Christmas shopping! I think I'm sending out Christmas cards on Thanksgiving. If the baby is not here by then! Hah! We're debating whether or not to get a real tree or a fake tree. I love a real tree, but I don't know if I want to bug with it this year, you know? If we get a fake tree we could set it up this weekend (just kidding!).

I think my dinner's getting cold. I'd better move my booty.

Halloween Was Fun

So it's done and over with! Dear stepson was so excited and so cute. We all had a fun time. It's the first time I've been the "adult" while trick-or-treating. It was fun though. I think I walked a mile. I definitely got my exercise last night!

Another holiday come and gone. :) I was sitting back eating a cupcake yesterday, and I realized- uh-oh... Here comes the food... Holiday parties and potlucks... It's my favorite time of the year. But I'm gonna get fat. Ugh. I guess all I can do is keep exercising and at least not become sedentary because I don't think avoiding all of the treats and goodies is feasible for me. I never pig-out completely, but I always like to try a little bit of this and a little bit of that. Oh well. I'll just have a lot of work ahead of me in the spring to get back into shape. I'm still slightly horrified at the idea of swapping my old body for a new one, complete with "Mommy butt"...

Enyway. Back to the kids. So, dear stepson had a great time. We didn't really stay out that long because his little feet were getting tired and it was really cold! He doesn't have a ton of candy, but I don't know what we're going to do with what he has! Maybe we should just go ahead and let him eat it and get the craziness over with. He had a fun time, so that's what's important. Last year we missed trick-or-treating with him because we were in Tennessee. He was really happy to have us there. And to end out the evening, he peed his pants! Now that's just an all-around good time for a 6-year-old, I think. He was having so much fun that either he didn't think about it, or he just couldn't take the time out to go... but eventually, it's gotta happen some way or another. I didn't say anything because I'm sure I did the same thing at some point or another when I was a kid.

And of course I had to ask Elijah what he was doing in there- if he was having fun. I think he was asleep during most of it, since I was walking around. When we sat down over at dear bf's uncle's house, Elijah was moving like crazy! I think he had fun. Next year, what am I going to dress him as? He'll be so cute! and he'll almost be walking... definitely old enough to smile and giggle and squeal. Old enough to know what candy is... oy...

2006-11-08 (33 weeks)

Lost a Pound

So I went to the doctor last night. Everything is looking good. I lost a pound! They were worried about me! I don't know. I haven't been sick or anything, and I've been eating just as much as I normally do, so I think I'm okay. I've just been getting around a little bit more. We've been busy busy busy. Monday we went Christmas shopping for a couple of hours, so I got some exercise walking around and around. Last night we went grocery shopping and that took forever, so I was walking around and around again. Saturday I took my future stepson to the mall to play some arcade games and we walked around the mall for quite a while just wasting time.

So, I'm up to 150 pounds. I think that's a good number. As long as I keep eating well and exercising. I started out at 119, so shouldn't 31 pounds be a healthy enough weight gain?

I need to get back to work. I'm sure there are a lot of things that I'm forgetting to write about, but oh well!

Family Pics and Sunday Dinner

So we had a busy little weekend. Dear bf had the weekend off so we did a lot of things. Saturday I went scrapbooking with my friends all day long. That was really fun but I didn't get a lot done!! I swear, I'll get like 2 pages done and then I can't decide what to do after that!! I need to work on it though, so it'll be ready to start putting in baby pics when the baby gets here. We'll see! I think I'll be done with it by the time Elijah is off to college! Oh well. So far I have the pages of how I met his dad and our time down in Tennessee. I still want to put info pages about me and his dad (like where we were born, etc.) pages of all the grandparents (Reminder to self to take pictures when I'm up at my dad's this weekend!) pages of his brother and pages of his aunts and his uncle. I think that's it and then it's onto the baby pages! I also want pages of my growing belly and how we found out we were pregnant and that type of stuff.

So dear bf was just a little bit miffed when I got home Saturday night around 5 or 6. He was perfectly fine before I left the house! But I guess once he started cleaning the kitchen and saw how bad it actually was, he kinda flipped out. Oh well! I kept telling him that it was piling up... I've been keeping up with it pretty well, I think, until this week when I got sick Wednesday night. But anyway. Basically from Wednesday night until Saturday morning nothing got done so it was kinda yucky. And he had company coming in, so he wasn't too pleased. He could have mentioned he was having company! Or he coulda asked me to come home earlier to help out. He's such a woman sometimes!

But he and his friend ended up having a good time anyway so he was in a better mood on Sunday. On Sunday he planned on having a big dinner with his dad. At the last minute he asked me to make some macaroni and cheese (homemade of course) and homemade mashed potatoes. The mashed potatoes turned out great, but the macaroni and cheese was like a nightmare! I tried to rush it, and ick! They all ate it, but I couldn't even stomach it! Ick!! It's never turned out *that* bad... whew! Oh well, hopefully I will be redeemed on Thanksgiving. But that's all I'm making. Mac and cheese and peach cobbler (perhaps). I don't know how you pregos that are making Thanksgiving dinner are gonna do it! That's a lot of work! I about fell over spending that 30 minutes in the kitchen with the mac and cheese, mashed potatoes and crescent rolls...

I gotta get back to work!

Anyway, oh yeah, we got our family pictures done and I got ripped off again!! I always do that! They always sell you on a cheap package, but you only get one pose! This time I was sure I asked whether or not I could get another pose at the cheap price if we decided we wanted it or whatever... She lied to me! She lied she lied she lied... and said that we could. The old bait and switch. She didn't put anything in writing, but I swear I asked in every way whether or not you could do that. Hmph. The last time was at Walmart and this lady was at Kmart and whenever we bought the package she went on and on about how bad Walmart was about that... and then she did the same thing to me. And when I got there on Sunday to take the pictures, she wasn't there and the people that were there were just shocked that she would say that to me. Whatever, people. Liars... all of them! :) They gave me a free 8x10 of one of the other poses for my "trouble". Then I ended up buying a sheet for 12.99 of me & dear bf with dear bf's hand on the belly. I wish I was rich enough to actually go to a decent place and get some professional ones done, you know? But that was our family pic story. Whenever the baby is born I might get a membership (I think that's what they do) at JcPenney or Target or Sears or someplace... I've got all kinds of coupons so I'm sure I could figure something out. 'Cause don't you need to do pictures like every 3 months when they are first born?

Okay. Back to work again.

Jobless!! And Thanksgiving Dinner...

So the law firm I was temping for got sick of seeing me waddle around the place and they went ahead and let me go. The good news is that my doctor was kind enough to sign me out of work. We'll see if they'll let me collect the short term disability I paid for. We'll see. I should have filed for it today, but I was soooo lazy today. It seems that now that I'm just sitting at home I am getting soooo lazy and exhausted. I think the baby is making his way downward and it is making me achy all over!

I can't wait for the "energy burst" that I'm supposed to have. We'll see! There's so much work to do. We've got to move our room around and move the crib and changing table in. I'm trying to wash all the baby clothes and sort though them to see what's what. I think mostly everything is NB or 0-3 month size, so let's hope that he's not bigger than normal. We'll see.

We're also going to cook Thanksgiving Dinner but I guess I'll talk about that later.

Thanksgiving Dinner!

We cooked dinner and it was really nice! We only had us and two other people, so it wasn't too taxing. And then one of our guests cleaned up! So that was cool.

I, myself, was responsible for rolls, macaroni and cheese and mashed potatoes. I figured out what went wrong with the mac and cheese the other day- the boys bought fat free cheese!! So, this time I bought the cheese and it went very well.

Um... I'm still trying to wash the baby clothes. I've been doing this for the past 2 months, I know. I actually have everything unpacked, un-hangered, and in a basket ready to go- to be washed. So. It's just a matter of doing it.

But anyway. Busy busy busy- I'd better go.

More Updates and Stuff

It has been a long week. My friend Syana came up for a visit yesterday and stayed the night. It was a whirlwind of cooking, eating and playing with the kids. Yesterday we went to the park, the mall to play games and bowling! It was craziness. Can you see my fat butt bowling. It was quite a sight. It was so weird too. I'm so used to dancing around and jumping up and down when I bowl- it was really weird because I couldn't exactly do that with how huge my belly is now.

Now I'm exhausted and I really need a nap. My friend just left at 2 and my future stepson's Grandma came and got him for lunch. :) I think she's keeping him for a few hours, so I should really take advantage of this time and take a nap. I wanted to catch up with this thing a little bit though since I never have time to write any more. That's kind of funny because I'm not working any more. I should have all the time in the world.

But I'm getting bigger and bigger and it's actually getting harder to move around. I wonder why some women get so many aches and pains and some women seemingly aren't bothered by pregnancy at all? It hardly seems fair. Maybe since my frame is so small the 30-some extra pounds are really weighing me down?

But I better get a move on this nap! I will try to write more later. I still haven't written about my visit up to my dad's last weekend or my latest doctor's appointment.

I bought Christmas cards!! I'm just waiting for our family pictures to come on Wednesday and those puppies are going out!

Homestretch!!!

Dear bf caught me talking to myself the other night, trying to get through a Braxton Hicks... He thinks I'm nuts. :) I was just laying there wiggling my pelvis, saying "move that baby down, move that baby down..."

Well? Baby needs to drop so we can get this show on the road! I am unconvinced that there is enough room in my pelvis for this big old baby. I wonder how long until we actually know that? The doctor said that if I don't go on my due date of Dec. 22nd, that she wants to induce on the 1st or 2nd of January. Oh no!! I thought I was having a Christmas baby!! I think I'm going on a jog around the block! I was talking to this other lady from a community outreach program here in town, and she said to ask my doctor if I could induce before the end of the year for tax purposes. :) I don't know. Sounds slightly frivolous- you know, like something Karma might get me for.

So, I'm going to try to get things going naturally. Somehow. But I remain unconvinced that there's room down there...

Dear bf was acting normal for the first time in weeks. He's been so nervous lately. Hopefully he's put that behind him. We shall see. I think it relaxed him to see me sit there and fold little baby clothes. I bought this baby detergent that smells soooo good. It smells just like a new baby... mmm mmm! I think they even put a dash of spit-up smell just to make it perfect.

So I finished the baby laundry!! I even separated out the too big clothes and put them up for when he grows.

Someone gave me a stack of preemie clothes that I don't think he'll be able to wear. I think he's already bigger than that. I don't know. We'll see. Now, I need to start my next project... eek! Right now I don't have any energy. I need to get moving. I know all this physical work will probably help "move that baby down" so that's extra motivation. Right now I think I'm going to go sit on the couch and watch some baby shows.

My next project is cleaning out my closet. It's not a huge project; I just need to move some crap out of there so I can move some other crap in there. Then we'll have room enough to move the bed over to the far wall and put the crib and changing table into our room.

I wonder how involved that changing table is? I've put together furniture before. I think dear bf would freak out if he came home and that was done!!

Anyway, I'd better get to watching TV so I can rest up and get ready for this next project.

2006-12-02 (37 weeks)

New Pics Posted

Well, I put some "new" pics up. :) They are from my shower on Sept. 30th. Just a little bit late, huh?

2006-12-09 (baby has arrived)

Baby's Here!!

I'll write more ASAP!

Birth Story

So I came to a conclusion just now. No matter how traumatizing my birth experience was... I still want more kids! I loved being pregnant and giving birth. Hopefully next time will go more smoothly! But Elijah is perfect. Perfect perfect perfect!! I promise to get pics on here ASAP.

It was any ordinary day. It was Tuesday night/Wednesday morning. I put dear bf's son into bed around 9 with his TV on and I fell asleep. I was still large and pregnant at the time. Hmm... So weird to be missing that big-old belly. I can't wait to have another one!! Around midnight dear bf comes in and shuts off his son's TV. Then he gets antsy and goes out again. His son starts to have a screaming fit. I try to get him to go to sleep, pleading, screaming and finally spanking. After an hour of this, he's still kicking and screaming and I catch a knee to the belly. I feel a contraction that feels like one of my Braxton Hicks and I lay down on my floor to catch my breath. I go into the bathroom and I notice that I am bleeding. I go into bf's son's room and turn on the TV and try to sleep. Yadda yadda yadda... a lot of other bad stuff happens. I call my doctor when they open (still bleeding) and they say to go into the emergency room. I get to the emergency room at 10:30 on Wednesday morning. All I had to eat was a bowl of cereal. I forget what we had for dinner Tuesday night. Luckily I had a hunch and I packed a bag for myself and the baby.

They admit me to the labor and delivery triage to start monitoring me. Some diabolical nurse "checks" me and I have never felt so much pain in my life! Maybe it was because I was sitting up and she rammed the spectulum up there? I don't know... But I started bawling because I knew that they would have to check me pretty often. I was completely effaced and a fingertip dialated. I think. A lot of my birth story is kind of fuzzy...

The bleeding had stopped around 8 am- (I filled about 6 or 7 pantiliners between 1am and 8am) and I think I started losing my mucus plug. They kept monitoring to make sure the placenta was not harmed and also since I'm Rh negative, they were worried that my blood mixed with the baby's (which turns out didn't matter because baby is A-). So they ran all of these tests. At first they were going to keep me for a few hours and then it was all day and finally they decided to keep me overnight.

I think the contraction monitor has a pain level of 10. :) It really digs in there! So, here I am, strapped to the bed (not literally- I think my mom freaked out when I said that!)... But they wouldn't allow me any mobility since the placenta was in danger. I couldn't even sit up because the monitor would fall out of place. I think they gave me some nubain for pain. I forget if they did that before or after I went into labor. That nubain made me looped out!! Apparently some people like that feeling, but I was miserable. I could still feel the pain but I was incoherent. I bet if I went in there now, those nurses would not even recognize me since I was so looped on drugs during my entire hospitalization. But man, it kinda sucked because here I am, still pregnant and every time I had to go to the bathroom I had to call a nurse to unhook me from the monitor. I tried to wait at least an hour every time. And I about cried one time when I was high on that nubain stuff because they were trying to convince me I had already gone.

I had like 3 different beds when I was there (4 if you count triage)! One regular bed, one delivery bed and one, I don't know... Some kind of exhibitionist forcep delivery bed...

I went into labor around 2 or 3am Thursday, Dec 7th. I quickly progressed to 5 centimeters despite being trapped in bed and high on nubain. They then gave me the epidural and I fell asleep. I woke up and was 10 centimeters.

We waited for a bit for the baby to come down and I listened to my Baby Needs Baroque cd (excellent classical cd) to gather my focus. It's got my favorite song ever- Pachabel's Canon in D minor on there. It's baby's favorite song too. As far as I can tell.

So I pushed for 30 minutes with no progress (in my eyes- the nurse said otherwise). The delivery nurse was convinced that I could do this, but I thought the baby was too big. I was horrified at the thought that they might let me push for 3 hours before they intervened. I just felt like I didn't know what I was doing. I tried acting like I was pushing a poop out, but I think the baby was blocking my pooper. They let me rest and then I was at it again. I was watching that clock like a hawk. I pushed for another hour and I hit the wall, ladies... I hit the wall. I was convinced that the baby was too large for me. The nurse kept saying that the baby was moving down but I was convinced he was trapped. I swear I tried I tried I really tried. I pushed, I wriggled and pushed. Maybe it was the epidural but I just wasn't feeling any progress. I was losing hope. I kept asking the nurses if they lost hope yet. I speculated on jumping out the window. Sadly, we were only 3 floors up, so I think I just would have broken a leg or something.

So I started crying. I know I know... I'm a wimp. But I hadn't eaten since god knows when. I hadn't had any sleep since god knows when. My adventure had started like Tuesday night and I'd been in the hospital since the previous morning. Oh and, my uterus was always contracting. To the point where the monitor didn't really work on me. So when they said push on a contraction, I was like, it's always a contraction!!

Anyway, I was crying and in severe pain. They decided to do the forceps. They topped off my epidural for the 2nd time but I didn't receive any relief because baby was in the birth canal. I heard one of the nurses or somebody say, well, judging from the death grip she has on the bed rail, I don't think she's getting any relief. :) I just shut my eyes and went to another place. I didn't feel the forceps. I just prayed that it would be over soon and I wouldn't be irreparably damaged and that baby would be okay. Like every one on the floor was in there. The doctor was sitting on a stool and they raised the bed to his eye level and shined the surgery spotlights right on, well, you know... There were like 20 people in there. I guess they never do forceps deliveries any more so every student nurse and intern on the floor was in there, wide-eyed. I didn't care at that point. They pulled the baby out and he was loopy too. He didn't really cry too much. He sat there and babbled to his grandmother (bf's mom) for like 30 minutes.

I was in complete and utter shock. I'm still in shock. I know he's mine and I know that I can't get enough of him. But this whole "mom" thing still soaking in.

But he's doing really well. We went to the doctor yesterday and thank god, he gained his weight back. He was born at 7-2 and Tuesday when the home visit nurse came by he was down to 6-11. The first night home from the hospital was very stressful. My milk hadn't come in yet and he couldn't sleep for more than 20 minutes at a time.

But right now the little one has been sleeping for 4 hours so I'm going to wake him up before he wakes up starving starving...

2006-12-19 (baby has arrived)

Baby Pics

This is all I have so far!

I just wanted to jot some things down so I remember. I was 153 pounds the day before I delivered so my total weight gain was 34 pounds. Bf's sister and mother helped me (along with bf) deliver the baby. They thought I was hilarious because they've never seen me act like that.

I bought a roll of film and I'm going to use it!

2007-03-31 (baby has arrived)

New Pic and Goodbye?

I just wanted to post a new pic of my little one on here. I guess I need to find another blog site!

It's been fabulous being a mom. I haven't done any journalling for the past 3 months, so I need to find somewhere I can start doing that. It's really been a blur. He already sleeps through the night, but those first 2 months when he wanted to wake up every 2 hours were really tough!

Breastfeeding is great. It took us a very long time (like 8 weeks) to figure out how to do it... so hang in there for you new moms!